P9-ELD-897

■

The Chiropractor's Self-Help Back and Body Book

■

Other Books by Samuel Homola

Bonesetting, Chiropractic, and Cultism

Backache: Home Treatment and Prevention

Muscle Training for Athletes

A Chiropractor's Treasury of Health Secrets

Secrets of Naturally Youthful Health and Vitality

Doctor Homola's Natural Health Remedies

Doctor Homola's Life-Extender Health Guide

Doctor Homola's Fat-Disintegrator Diet

Peter Lupus' Guide to Radiant Health and Beauty: Mission Possible for Women (with Peter Lupus)

Peter Lupus' Celebrity Body Book—A Body-Improvement Guide for Men and Women (with Peter Lupus)

Doctor Homola's Macro-Nutrient Diet for Quick, Permanent Weight Loss

Inside Chiropractic: A Patient's Guide

Dedicated to rational chiropractors who recognize their limitations and to those health-care professionals whose cooperation enables us all to do what is best for the patient

ORDERING

Trade bookstores in the United States and Canada please contact:

Publishers Group West
1700 Fourth Street, Berkeley CA 94710
Phone: (800) 788-3123   Fax: (510) 528-3444

Hunter House books are available at bulk discounts for textbook course adoptions; to qualifying community, health-care, and government organizations; and for special promotions and fund-raising. For details please contact:

Special Sales Department
Hunter House Inc., PO Box 2914, Alameda CA 94501-0914
Phone: (510) 865-5282   Fax: (510) 865-4295
E-mail: ordering@hunterhouse.com

Individuals can order our books from most bookstores, by calling **(800) 266-5592,** or from our website at **www.hunterhouse.com**

The Chiropractor's Self-Help Back and Body Book

Your *Complete* Guide to Relieving Aches and Pains at Home and on the Job

■

Samuel Homola, D.C.

Line drawings by Bibiana Neal

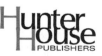

Hunter House PUBLISHERS

Gen Fund 9/02 18⁰⁰

Copyright © 2002 by Samuel Homola, D.C.

All rights reserved. No part of this publication may be reproduced or transmitted in any form or by any means, electronic or mechanical, including photocopying and recording, or introduced into any information storage and retrieval system without the written permission of the copyright owner and the publisher of this book. Brief quotations may be used in reviews prepared for inclusion in a magazine, newspaper, or for broadcast. For further information please contact:

Hunter House Inc., Publishers
PO Box 2914
Alameda CA 94501-0914

LIBRARY OF CONGRESS CATALOGING-IN-PUBLICATION DATA

Homola, Samuel.
   The chiropractor's self-help back and body book : your complete guide to relieving common aches and pains at home and on the job / Samuel Homola; line drawings by Bibiana Neal.-- 1st ed.
      p. cm.
Includes index.
ISBN 0-89793-377-X (cl) -- ISBN 0-89793-376-1 (pb)
1. Backache--Popular works. 2. Chiropractic--Popular works. 3. Pain--Popular works. 4. Self-care, Health. I. Title.
RD771.B217 H655 2002
617.5'6406--dc21   2002068687

PROJECT CREDITS

Cover Design: Peri Poloni, Knockout Books
Book Production: Hunter House; Interior Design: Jinni Fontana
Copy Editor: Debbie Epstein; Editorial Assistance: Rachel E. Bernstein
Proofreader: John David Marion
Indexer: Nancy D. Peterson
Acquisitions Editor: Jeanne Brondino
Editor: Alexandra Mummery
Publicity Coordinator: Earlita K. Chenault
Sales and Marketing Coordinator: JoAnne Retzlaff
Customer Service Manager: Christina Sverdrup
Order Fulfillment: Lakdhon Lama
Administrator: Theresa Nelson
Computer Support: Peter Eichelberger
Publisher: Kiran S. Rana

Printed and Bound by Transcontinental Printing in Canada

9 8 7 6 5 4 3 2 1   First Edition   02 03 04 05 06

▪ Contents ▪

List of Illustrations   x

Foreword. xiii

Preface: How to Use This Book. xiv

Introduction: What This Book Can Do for You.   1

1 ▪ Pinpointing the Cause of Your Head, Neck, Shoulder, Arm, Back,
    and Leg Pain   4
    How to Get the Help You Need   4
    Distinguishing Type O from Type M Disorders   6
    Classifying Your Headache   6
    How to Determine the Cause of Your Neck, Shoulder, and Arm Pain. . . . 10
    How to Analyze Back, Hip, and Leg Pain 14
    Ten Tests for Type M Back Pain 25
    Solutions for Your Problems 28

2 ▪ Headache: Home Treatment and Prevention 30
    Self-Help with Home Remedies. 31
    Simple Techniques to Relieve Tension Headaches 32
    How to Use Rest and Relaxation to Relieve Tension Headaches. 36
    How to Relieve Head Pain with an Ice Pack 37
    Coffee and Cigarettes Constrict Blood Vessels. 38
    Alcohol and Headache. 39
    Headache-Causing Amines in Wine and Cheese 39
    Hot Dog Headaches. 39
    Too Much Salt Can Cause Headaches 41
    An Elimination Diet for Cluster and Migraine Headaches 41
    Environmental Causes of Headaches. 42
    Exercise as a Treatment for Headache 43
    How to Relieve the Headache of Hypoglycemia. 44
    The Triangle of Constipation, Headache, and Backache 46
    When You Need Medication 51

3 ■ How to Relieve Neck, Shoulder, and Arm Pain **53**

The Different Sources of Neck Pain 54

How to Handle the Common Neck Crick. 54

Slipped Discs and Pinched Nerves 60

How to Relieve Neck and Arm Pain by Stretching Your Neck at Home . . 63

Home Care for Shoulder Bursitis, Arthritis, and Tendonitis. 66

When Elbow Pain Occurs 69

Special Wrist and Hand Problems. 71

4 ■ What You Can Do about Back, Hip, and Leg Pain **75**

Time Is on Your Side!. 76

It's Probably Only a Strain. 76

Red Flags Indicating Possible Spinal Cancer 78

Bed Rest for Acute Back Pain 78

Relieving Back Pain with Pillows 81

Moving Around on Crutches. 83

Choosing Between Heat and Cold 83

Constipation Caused by Back Pain 84

When You Need a Back Support 84

Disc Problems and the Types of Pain They Cause. 85

How to Use Traction at Home to Relieve Back and Leg Pain 92

Dealing with Structural Abnormalities. 96

How Spinal Curvatures Cause Back Pain 96

How to Handle Common Low-Back Joint Deformities 100

Prevention and Treatment for Osteoporosis (Brittle Vertebrae) 103

Strengthen Your Back Bones and Your Back Muscles
    with Special Exercises 112

Can Stress Cause Backache? 114

Manipulation Versus Medication 115

**5 ■ How You Can Loosen and Align Your Spinal Joints
Safely and Effectively** **119**

The Mystery of Cracking Joints. 120

Spinal Care Without Fear. 121

Prevention Is Your Responsibility! 122

Stretching Ankle, Thigh, Hip, and Back Muscles 124

How to Loosen Your Vertebrae 130

Back Massage at Home 137

6 ■ How to Eat to Reduce Body Weight and Relieve Backache **140**

Dieting Can Make You Fat! 141

Healthy Diets and Calorie Reduction 142

Get Rid of Backache by Getting Rid of Your Potbelly 143

The New High-Fiber, High-Carbohydrate Reducing Diet 144

How to Balance Your Diet 145

The Healthful Benefits of Fiber Supplied by Natural Carbohydrates 147

Basic Rules for Losing Weight 148

A Sample Low-Fat, Low-Calorie Natural Foods Diet Plan 151

How to Determine Your Calorie Requirement 153

How to Balance Energy Nutrients 157

Two Sample Balanced Calorie-Counting Reducing Diets 158

You Can Eat Heartily with Natural Foods! 160

The Selection and Preparation of Foods Is Important 161

7 ■ Protective and Remedial Exercise in a Personalized

Back-Care Program **164**

Exercise Is an Important Preventive Measure 165

Begin Your Exercise Program with Abdominal Exercises 168

Strengthening the Supporting Muscles on the Back of Your Spine 170

Strengthen Your Legs to Protect Your Back 174

Strengthen Your Entire Body 175

Strengthen Back Muscles with One Barbell Exercise 176

Aiding Exercise with Water 177

What to Do about Postural Kyphosis 177

It Takes Time to Develop Back Muscles 179

8 ■ How to Handle Spinal Arthritis in a Self-Help Program **182**

Common Forms of Spinal Arthritis 182

Arthritis Treatment and Prevention at Home 183

Self-Help in the Care of Wear-and-Tear Osteoarthritis (OA) 185

How to Cope with Inflammatory Rheumatoid Arthritis (RA) 190

The Bamboo Spine of Ankylosing Spondylitis (AS) 193

Gouty Arthritis and Backache 196

Myofascitis and Other Muscle Problems 198

Sleeping with Arthritis 200

A Firm Mattress, Sex, and Other Remedies 200

Systemic Lupus Erythematosus (SLE): The Great Pretender 201

**9 ■ How to Prevent Back Strain by Using Proper Sitting,
Standing, Lifting, and Sleeping Postures** **203**

Protect Your Spinal Curves with Good Posture 204

A Simple Rule for Maintaining Good Standing Posture 205

The Special Problems of Sitting 209

How to Protect Your Spine with Proper Lifting Techniques 212

How to Protect Your Back with Proper Sleeping Postures 214

Postural Hypotension 218

Ergonomics: Posture Problems at Work 218

10 ■ Preventing and Easing Back Pain During Pregnancy **222**

Prenatal Prevention Measures 223

Relieving Back Pain During Pregnancy 225

Postpartum Problems 226

Backache Relief with Moist Heat and Massage 229

Keep in Touch with Your Doctor 229

11 ■ How to Protect a Painful Back During Sex and while Pregnant . . . **231**

The Benefits of a Healthy Sex Life 232

The Special Problems of Pregnancy and Menopause 233

Sex with a Bad Back 234

12 ■ Evaluating Back and Leg Pain after Middle Age **240**

The Many Causes of Back and Leg Pain 241

What Is Causing Your Leg Pain 242

The Question of Cancer 243

What about Kidney Stones? 243

Osteoporosis as a Cause of Back Pain 244

13 ■ When You Need the Help of a Specialist **248**

Specialists in a Nutshell 249

The Specialty of Family Practice 250

Orthopedists and Neurosurgeons 252

Physiatrists and Rehabilitation 252

Internists: The Diagnosticians 253

Radiology: X-ray Specialists 253

Rheumatologists: The Arthritis Doctors 253

Osteopaths: Diversified Doctors 254

Chiropractors as Back Specialists 254
Physical Therapists and Body Care 256
Last-Resort Surgical Remedies for Back Problems 257

14 ■ Sense and Nonsense in Chiropractic Care of Back Pain 259
Finding a Chiropractic Back Specialist 260
How to Avoid Questionable Chiropractors 261
Doctors Must Work Together 266

15 ■ Questions Patients Commonly Ask about Back Trouble 268

Endnotes 279

Glossary 280

Index 291

▪ List of Illustrations ▪

Fig. 1-1   Shoulder pain caused by attempting to scratch your back
may be a sign of a mechanical-type shoulder problem 12

Fig. 1-2   The spine is a complicated stack of bones held together by
ligaments and interlocking joints 18

Fig. 1-3   Symptoms aggravated by straight-leg raising may be indicative of
nerve root entrapment 26

Fig. 1-4   "Figure-4" testing is positive for a hip socket problem when
pain or locking prevents lowering of the knee 27

Fig. 2-1   A simple resistive neck exercise that will strengthen neck
muscles and help maintain a normal cervical curve 43

Fig. 3-1   Fluffing up the bottom edge of a thin pillow so that the back
of the neck and the back of the head are equally supported . . . 59

Fig. 3-2   Simple neck stretching at home using a cervical traction
harness to relieve neck, shoulder, and arm pain 64

Fig. 3-3   A shoulder pulley exercise used to restore or improve range
of motion in a stiff or painful shoulder. 69

Fig. 4-1   Relieving back pain by placing a pillow under the knees to
relieve tension on hip flexors and prevent arching of the spine . 81

Fig. 4-2   Using a sofa to provide traction that may help relieve lower
back and leg pain 82

Fig. 4-3   Leg pain caused by disc herniation or spur formation in the
lower back 86

Fig. 4-4   Areas where pain, numbness, and other symptoms are
commonly felt when spinal nerves are pinched or irritated 87

Fig. 4-5   Low-back traction to relieve sciatic leg pain that is not
relieved by lying down 94

Fig. 4-6   A hump is apparent on one side of the back when you bend
forward if scoliosis is present 97

Fig. 4-7   Spondylolisthesis, or forward slipping of a vertebra, most
commonly occurs in the lower back 101

Fig. 4-8   Appearance of a hump in the upper back of a postmenopausal
woman may signal the presence of a collapsed vertebra 104

Fig. 4-9   Straight-arm pullovers with a throw cushion under the upper back will combat thoracic slumping 113

Fig. 5-1   Bending forward to stretch tight hamstrings without placing pressure on the intervertebral discs 126

Fig. 5-2   Bent-knee sit-ups to strengthen abdominal muscles without placing excessive leverage on the lumbar spine 128

Fig. 5-3   Arching your back while on your hands and knees to warm up muscles and loosen vertebrae 131

Fig. 5-4   Lying over a roll of carpet will loosen and extend the thoracic spine. 132

Fig. 5-5   A supine low-back twist stretches tight back muscles and loosens lumbar vertebrae. 134

Fig. 7-1   Muscles on both sides of the trunk are important for supporting the spine 166

Fig. 7-2   The tripod leg-extension exercise stretches hip flexors and strengthens back and hip muscles 170

Fig. 7-3   This prone back-arching exercise strengthens muscles up and down the back 173

Fig. 7-4   The supine bridge exercise strengthens muscles in the back, hips, and legs without uncomfortable strain 174

Fig. 7-5   Shrugging the shoulders while holding a weight at arm's length will strengthen shoulder girdle muscles 178

Fig. 8-1   An infrared heat lamp can be used to heat a warm, moist towel to be applied over any arthritic joint 184

Fig. 9-1   Bad posture, in addition to causing chronic back pain, can detract from physical appearance 205

Fig. 9-2   Placing one foot on a low stool during prolonged standing will relieve strain on the lower back 208

Fig. 9-3   Sit with chair height adjusted so that your thighs and lower legs are at right angles when both feet are flat on the floor 211

Fig. 9-4   Keep your back flat and as vertical as possible while using your legs to lift a heavy weight 212

Fig. 9-5   The increasing use of computers at home and on the job requires special attention to sitting postures 219

Fig. 10-1 The basin of a female pelvis is wider than that of a male pelvis; the sacroiliac joints further relax during birth 223

Fig. 10-2   Supporting body weight between two chairs, both feet on the floor, decompresses joints and discs in the lower spine 226

Fig. 10-3   Holding a baby, or any weight, with the arms extended places damaging leverage on the lower back 227

Fig. 10-4   A doctor might prescribe a special maternity corset when there is low-back pain during pregnancy 228

Fig. 11-1   A male with back pain can be a passive sexual partner while lying on his back 236

Fig. 11-2   The side posture position allows penetration from behind when a female is pregnant or has back trouble 237

Fig. 11-3   The "doggy position" is safe when the female is pregnant or has back trouble 237

Fig. 11-4   This supported position at the edge of the bed can be helpful during pregnancy 238

Fig. 14-1   The pinching of a nerve occurs when there is disc herniation, spur formation, thickening of ligaments or cartilage, or some other pathological process 263

Important Note

The material in this book is intended to provide a review of self-help treatment for common aches and pains. Every effort has been made to provide accurate and dependable information. However, you should be aware that professionals in the field may have differing opinions, and change is always taking place. If any of the treatments described herein are used, they should be undertaken only under the guidance of a licensed health-care practitioner. The author, editors, and publishers cannot be held responsible for any error, omission, professional disagreement, outdated material, or adverse outcomes that derive from use of any of these treatments in a program of self-care or under the care of a licensed practitioner.

▪ Foreword ▪

It's always a good idea to see your family physician before attempting self-help for relief of pain. But once a diagnosis has been made and any need for medical care has been satisfied, self-help is often useful and sometimes essential in relieving and preventing pain. This book by Samuel Homola, D.C., carefully describes and outlines mechanical-type problems that can benefit from self-help, such as home remedies, ergonomics, and behavior modification. He is also careful to steer readers away from the fads and the nonsense commonly associated with health advice offered in popular publications.

Dr. Homola's reputation as a rational, science-based chiropractor is reflected in the caveats he offers to persons seeking advice about health and health-care practitioners.

In this age of computers and electronic media, people are more knowledgeable than ever about health and treatment methods. Physicians expect to be questioned by their patients. Just about everyone is seeking information through online computer websites. Everyone can, and should, make an effort to seek the information needed to relieve pain and build good health.

This new book by Dr. Homola offers self-help advice that separates sense from nonsense. It may be one of the most useful, comprehensive, and scientifically reliable books of its type, offering advice for lay persons who want to do all they can to help themselves in the treatment and prevention of many common aches and pains, especially back pain.

The Chiropractor's Complete Self-Help Back and Body Book would be a useful addition to every home health library.

— **E.A. (Jack) Gedosh, M.D.**

▪ Preface ▪
How to Use This Book

With the instructions offered in this book, you'll learn how to recognize the various types of back trouble and what to do about them. You'll also learn about the various tests used to diagnose back trouble and how to perform many of them yourself.

If you need the help of a specialist, this book will be a useful guide in selecting the type of specialist needed. And to make sure you are well informed about what medical science has to offer, you'll be provided with some basic information about new and effective methods of diagnosing and treating back trouble.

If you read and follow the instructions outlined in this book, you'll be able to do more for your back than anyone—including your doctor. And you'll be less likely to ever need back surgery. As a chiropractor with forty years of experience treating back trouble, I can tell you without reservation that most forms of back trouble are preventable. I can assure you that time and self-help can be just as important as the most expensive therapy in treating most forms of back trouble. Use of ice packs or moist heat at home, for example, can be as effective as the most expensive physical therapy. This book is filled with simple remedies that can be used safely and effectively at home.

If you want to take control of your back trouble, get a diagnosis from your family physician or an orthopedic specialist and then use this book to do all you can to help yourself. (Keep in touch with your doctor, however, so that you quickly obtain medical help if you need it.)

Remember that your back is *your* responsibility. If you don't take care of it, no one else will. A good book on back care, such as the one you now have in your hands, will help you prevent incapacitating back pain. Study this book carefully and keep it handy for reference so that you can stay out of the ranks of the suffering, disabled, and unemployed back patients.

Every chapter in this book covers a different subject related to the treatment and prevention of back pain and other mechanical-type problems. All of these chapters together add up to a complete program of self-help for common aches and pains. Most people will turn to the chapter that interests them most, seeking immediate relief for their specific pain. But it's important to first determine if medical attention is needed and if there is a problem that could benefit from self-help.

Chapter 1, "Pinpointing the Cause of Your Head, Neck, Arm, Back, and Leg Pain," tells how to distinguish simple mechanical-type (Type M) problems from the more serious organic (Type O) problems that should be brought to the attention of a physician. Everyone should read this very important chapter before deciding on a diagnosis and a method of treatment.

Headaches are very common and are often related to neck tension. There are many causes of headache, however, some of which can be serious. Chapter 2 describes the various types of headaches that exist and offers home treatment and prevention tips that can be used on their own or along with any treatment your physician might prescribe.

Shoulder and arm pain are often the results of a neck problem. Chapter 3 is devoted entirely to the various causes of neck, shoulder, and arm pain, offering specific measures designed to correct and relieve each type of problem, ranging from neck traction that can be used at home to the use of a pulley exercise that helps restore normal movement in a "frozen" shoulder.

Chapter 4, "What You Can Do about Back, Hip, and Leg Pain," covers the most common problem of all—back pain and its associated problems, such as leg pain. Once bone disease and other serious problems have been ruled out, self-help, such as use of exercise and hot or cold packs, is absolutely essential in the treatment and prevention of back pain. Everyone should be aware of the various causes of back pain and what to do about them. Even if you have osteoporosis or scoliosis, there is much you can do to help yourself. Self-examination tips will help determine what kind of back or leg pain you have.

Spinal manipulation provided by a health-care professional is sometimes helpful in relieving back pain. But when you are simply sore and stiff, there are some back-loosening techniques described in Chapter 5 that can be done safely and effectively at home.

We all know that excess body weight can overload joints and aggravate back pain as well as contribute to the development of a variety of health problems. Chapter 6 outlines a natural foods diet regimen that will improve health as well as reduce body weight. Everyone should read this chapter, even if they are not overweight and do not have back pain.

Exercise is an important part of any program designed to relieve back pain and reduce body weight, but not everyone can or should do the same exercises. Chapter 7 tells how to use exercise to prevent back trouble and to relieve some types of back pain. If you have spinal arthritis, you'll want to read Chapter 8, which offers special instructions in the use of exercise and other measures designed to relieve inflammation, stiffness, and pain.

No matter what type of back trouble or arthritis you might have, or even if you have no problems at all, it's important to use good posture in everything you do. Improper lifting is a common cause of back strain. Bad sitting and sleeping postures can lead to back trouble or aggravate a bad back. Chapter 9 tells you everything you need to know about how to protect your back and arthritic joints with good postures.

Some types of back pain fall into special categories, such as back pain during pregnancy (Chapter 10), back pain during sex (Chapter 11), and back pain associated with the aging process (Chapter 12). These chapters offer special instructions for those who need special help with some of these problems—if not now, maybe sometime in the future.

Although self-help is an essential part of any treatment program for mechanical-type problems, any persistent or unrelieved pain should be brought to the attention of a specialist. Chapter 13 discusses the various medical specialties that handle the type of problems discussed in this book and offers suggestions on how to determine what kind of specialist you should see. Many people go to a chiropractor when they have back pain. There are different types of chiropractors, some of whom use unscientific treatment methods. Chapter 14 discusses some of the controversial aspects of chiropractic and offers suggestions for finding a good, ethical practitioner.

Chapter 15 contains a number of commonly asked questions as well as simple answers that will ease the fear and confusion of back pain victims who are seeking information. The glossary at the back of this book will define many of the terms and procedures encountered when seeking treatment for back pain.

— **Samuel Homola, D.C.**

■

The Chiropractor's
Self-Help Back
and Body Book

■

▪ Introduction ▪
What This Book Can Do for You

Back pain is one of our most common ailments. At least 90 percent of us will experience some form of back or neck pain during our lifetime. The most common age of patients suffering from acute back pain falls between the ages of thirty and fifty-five. This is when the spinal discs begin to deteriorate from wear and tear—a time when the individual is most productive as a wage earner.

According to the Agency for Healthcare Research and Quality of the U.S. Public Health Service, low-back trouble is the most common cause of disability among persons under the age of forty-five. In the general population as a whole, low-back problems are the second most common reason for office visits to primary care physicians and the most common reason for office visits to orthopedic surgeons, neurosurgeons, and occupational medicine physicians. Low-back problems have been described as the third most common reason for surgery performed in the United States.[1] In 1999, the Centers for Disease Control and Prevention reported that one in five Americans had a disabling health problem, 16.5 percent of whom had back or spine problems.

A variety of symptoms involving other parts of the body—including the head, shoulders, arms, hips, and legs—are also often associated with back and spinal problems. Tension headache, for example, commonly accompanies neck trouble, low-back problems often cause hip and leg pain, and so on. The same treatment used to relieve neck and back pain that involves spinal structures will therefore often relieve pain, numbness, tingling, and other symptoms that occur in other parts of the body.

The spine consists of 103 joints and 23 discs connecting 26 vertebrae to the skull, ribs, and pelvis, supported by layers of muscles, ligaments, and tendons (see the Glossary for the definitions of these terms). There are also

31 pairs of spinal nerves that pass between vertebrae, supplying musculoskeletal structures in every portion of the body. With so many parts, it's not surprising that back pain and neck pain are so common. Unfortunately, it's sometimes difficult to distinguish back-related problems from more serious organic diseases. For this reason, it's always important to see a doctor in order to determine what is causing your aches and pains, especially when they are acute (severe or have been present for less than three months) or when they persist for more than a few weeks.

Keep in mind, however, that a doctor can help you with only a small percentage of your back problems. Most of what must be done in back care must be done by you. Once your doctor has ruled out organic disease and identified your problem, there are many things you can do to help yourself. In most cases, a simple back strain will resolve itself in two to four weeks if there is no previous history of back trouble. Back trouble does tend to be chronic, however, so any program of back care should be a long-range procedure—a personal, carefully planned lifelong program. And the more you know about the diagnosis and treatment of back pain, the more you can do about relieving your pain and speeding your recovery.

The low back or lumbar area of the spine, where disc herniation most commonly occurs, is the site of most back pain. Fortunately, simple strain and degenerative changes are the most common causes of low-back pain. Neck (cervical spine) pain is nearly as common as low-back pain, and, like the lumbar spine, is often a site of disc herniation. The thoracic spine (the portion of the spine between the shoulder blades) rarely presents symptoms of disc herniation, since the discs in this area are thinner and the vertebrae are stabilized by the attachment of ribs. So most of the time, except in cases where there is advanced osteoporosis or osteoarthritis, the trouble will be in the neck or low back. Because of the greater amount of movement in the cervical and lumbar portions of the spine, there is a greater probability of disc herniation and degenerative changes with spur formation in these areas of the spine. After a correct diagnosis has been made, you'll be able to help yourself in the care of these problems.

Spinal manipulation provided by a good chiropractor is sometimes helpful in the treatment of some types of back pain. Your family doctor might refer you to a physical therapist who uses a variety of treatment modalities. When pain persists or radiates down an arm or a leg, you should seek referral to an orthopedist or a neurologist who can offer a more definitive diagnosis based on high-tech diagnostic procedures.

Fortunately, most neck and back problems will be of the mechanical-type variety, which can benefit from the self-help procedures outlined in this book. This book is not just about neck and back trouble, however; it covers a variety of mechanical-type aches and pains and many other problems that are often associated with back trouble. Using this book as a guide, you can determine what your problem is, what you can do to help yourself, and who you should see when you need professional help.

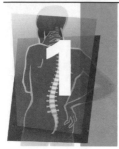

Pinpointing the Cause of Your Head, Neck, Shoulder, Arm, Back, and Leg Pain

If you are one of the millions of Americans suffering from back or neck pain, it will not surprise you to learn that headache, arm or leg pain, and other common aches and pains are often associated with a neck or back problem. There is plenty that you can do to help yourself, but before you begin by turning to the chapter that interests you most, you should read the self-exam checklists outlined in this chapter. These include things you and your doctor can do to rule out organic disease or a serious mechanical problem. If you have fever, persistent pain, or some other alarming symptoms, for example, or if you have suffered a painful injury, you should, of course, see a doctor immediately. However, once the diagnosis has been made and if it has been established that you have a simple mechanical problem, you may begin the appropriate self-help program.

How to Get the Help You Need

Clyde T. visited my office complaining of recurring pain in his back, hip, and leg. "The pain goes away when I lie down," he explained, "but it comes back when I stand for a while or when I sit for a long time. Leaning over to work on my car really makes my back hurt."

An office examination and a case history revealed that Clyde had a low-back structural abnormality that had been strained by using bad posture while changing a tire on his car. With time and a few simple home treatments, Clyde's back and leg pain disappeared. He was also instructed in the correct postures and lifting techniques described in Chapter 9, making it less likely that he would suffer a recurrence of back pain.

Sixty-year-old Debra D. also had back and leg pain. "I have sciatica," she told friends. "My mother had it and now I have it. I can treat it myself with a poultice, just as my mother did." But Debra's leg pain, a radiation of nerve symptoms into her calf and foot, did not get better; it got worse. Her leg hurt constantly, twenty-four hours a day. Nothing seemed to relieve the pain. After months of suffering, Debra finally came in for an examination. It quickly became apparent that her leg pain was not coming from her spine, which is where sciatica pain comes from. Everything in her leg seemed normal. Deep tendon reflexes in her knees and ankles were normal, and her ankle pulse was strong, indicating a good flow of blood to her leg. The straight-leg-raise test, which you'll learn about later in this chapter, was negative. There wasn't anything to suggest that her leg pain was originating in the spine or leg. Even though her back hurt, she could move and bend without difficulty.

An X-ray examination of Debra's lumbar spine revealed a dangerously large abdominal aneurysm caused by stretching and splitting in the walls of the aortic artery! She was immediately referred to a surgeon who patched the ballooning aorta. Had the aneurysm gone undetected much longer, it could have ruptured, resulting in a fatal loss of blood.

If Debra had known a little more about how to distinguish mechanical disorders from organic problems, she would have been alerted to the possibility that her leg pain might be coming from somewhere other than her back.

As a general rule, anytime you have pain that radiates down an arm or a leg, you should not delay in seeing a doctor. Simple low-back pain on movement is usually not a cause for alarm. But when you have radiation down one of your legs, you might have referred pain from a herniated disc or some other serious problem that must be differentiated from an even more serious vascular disorder that might require immediate medical attention.

You should never attempt to replace a physician's expertise with amateur doctoring. You should, however, possess enough knowledge about your body and your back to help you decide when to help yourself and when to see a doctor. This book will provide you with the guidance you need to make the right decision in caring for your neck and back pain, so that you can help yourself and your doctor.

Distinguishing Type O from Type M Disorders

Whether you treat yourself or are treated by your doctor, it is absolutely essential that you determine whether you are suffering from a Type O or Type M problem. Type O problems involve infectious or organic disease, which should always be brought to the attention of a physician. Type M problems are mechanical in nature and involve muscles, joints, and ligaments. If pain is relieved by rest and increased by bending, getting in and out of a car, turning over in bed, when you cough or sneeze, or during any activity that places stress on your lower back, then your trouble is probably mechanical or Type M in nature.

A Type M problem, once diagnosed by a physician, almost always involves self-help and must often be treated at home. It goes without saying, of course, that when pain or symptoms persist or grow worse despite all you do to help yourself, regardless of the type of problem, you should see your doctor.

Classifying Your Headache

Since headache is nearly as prevalent as backache and often stems from neck trouble, let's start at the top and begin with your head in evaluating your aches and pains.

About 90 percent of all chronic headaches are the tension and migraine variety, which can usually be handled at home. Any headache can be a potentially serious symptom, however, and should not be regarded lightly when it is persistent or accompanied by certain signs. Headache accompanied by vomiting or visual disturbances, for example, should be brought to the attention of a neurologist. Headache accompanied by fever is usually a sign of infection.

Headaches that occur only during menstruation, after drinking alcohol, after eating certain foods, or while sitting in a stuffy room have obvious temporary causes. Most of us recognize a sinus headache because nasal congestion or blocked drainage cause pain above our eyes or over our cheekbones. A headache that occurs after being exposed to glaring light or following eye strain usually does not alarm us.

When a pregnant woman develops a sudden headache or when a child has a headache that is associated with fever or a stiff neck, we become concerned. And when a headache occurs following a head injury, it's important to call a doctor immediately.

Common sense often helps us determine whether a headache is serious or not. Any headache accompanied by unusual symptoms should alert us to the possibility of a serious problem.

About seven of every ten headaches are caused by simple tension that often originates in the muscles and joints of the neck. Doctors often refer to this type of headache as a "muscle contraction headache." If you suffer from this type of headache, as most of us do, you'll be able to help yourself with some of the remedies outlined in Chapter 2. Before you begin a self-help program for headache, however, you should familiarize yourself with some of the symptoms that accompany the various types of headaches.

Type O Headaches Caused by Organic Disease

The most serious types of headaches other than those resulting from head injury are those caused by brain tumors, aneurysms, and other diseases that place pressure on the brain. A persistent, progressive headache accompanied by vomiting, weakness on one side of the body, convulsions, mental changes, or disturbances in speech or sight should be investigated immediately by a neurologist. Such symptoms could indicate a serious problem.

If you have a persistent headache or any of the symptoms mentioned above, see your doctor. If a neurological examination is required, it might include such special tests as a lumbar puncture, an arteriogram, or a magnetic resonance imaging (MRI) study of the brain. A lumbar puncture is a spinal tap used to test the contents and pressure of the spinal fluids that circulate around the brain. In an arteriogram, a contrast agent (dye) is injected into the arteries so that the arteries in and around the brain can be visualized with X rays, computerized tomography (CT), or magnetic resonance imaging (MRI). A CT scan uses X rays, while an MRI uses magnetic energy that does not involve radiation.

Headache associated with fever could be the result of disease or infection. Meningitis (an inflammation of the membranes covering the brain and spinal cord), for example, would be suspected when fever, vomiting, or other symptoms are accompanied by a stiff neck. Kidney infection is usually accompanied by fever that causes a headache. I frequently see patients in my office who complain of backache and headache, but do not know that they have a fever caused by kidney infection.

You'll learn in Chapter 2 how a simple stiff neck caused by arthritis or tight neck muscles can cause tension headache. When headache is accompanied by fever, however, you cannot assume that you are suffering from a simple tension or muscle contraction headache, no matter how tight your neck is. So be on guard and take your temperature.

Pain alone is not a reliable sign in judging the seriousness of a headache. Some severe headaches, such as Type O migraine and cluster vascular headaches, are extremely painful but not serious in their effect on your health. A more serious and potentially fatal brain tumor may be less painful than a simple tension headache since brain tissue does not have pain fibers. Pain may not be severe until expansion of the tumor produces pressure inside the skull. Headaches that come and go and last only a few hours or a few days are usually not serious and are most often of the tension and migraine variety. If you have high blood pressure and you develop a sudden, severe headache accompanied by drowsiness or muscular weakness, your doctor might want to examine you for a brain hemorrhage. A drooping eyelid and a stiff neck might mean that a blood vessel has broken in the membranes that cover your brain. Once again, however, these are unusual symptoms that should alert you and your doctor to the possibility that you might be suffering from something more serious that a simple tension headache.

Temporal arteritis, infection and inflammation of blood vessels on one or both sides of the head, may be mistaken for migraine and can lead to such serious complications as stroke or blindness. This Type O disease is often associated with polymyalgia, or aching and stiffness in muscles, and may be detected in an early stage only by the most observant physician.

The Puzzle of Migraine Headache

Migraine headaches are recurring systemic headaches that are preceded by visual disturbances and are accompanied by nausea or vomiting. Although the cause of migraine is often not known, this type of headache is usually so severe that a neurological examination should be done to rule out organic disease. Migraines usually recur despite all you do to prevent them. Blood chemical changes that constrict or dilate blood vessels to trigger migraine can be caused by such everyday factors as low blood sugar or a food protein (such as amines) in susceptible persons.

Some less severe migraine and pseudomigraine headaches that resemble migraine can be relieved with simple home remedies. In the case of classic migraine, however, special drugs, such as an ergotamine derivative, can be used to relieve severe pain by constricting dilated blood vessels. However, such drugs must be prescribed by a physician who has correctly diagnosed your headache.

Recognizing a Cluster Headache

Not much is known about the cause of cluster headaches. They occur primarily in men and are the most painful of all headaches. Fortunately, this type of headache is not common, affecting less than 1 percent of the population. A cluster headache, like a migraine, is a systemic vascular response to a variety of factors, ranging from stress to food chemicals, that trigger constriction and then dilation of blood vessels around the brain.

When cluster headaches occur, there is usually severe pain on one side of the head, along with a runny nose and a watery eye on the side with the pain. Although this type of headache is often diagnosed as a sinus problem, it may, in fact, be another form of vascular headache, much like migraine. There may be short, severe attacks of pain lasting twenty minutes to three hours, occurring two or three times a day for as long as four to six weeks. The pain of cluster headaches is so severe that the sufferer may have to rely upon a physician for prescription medication.

If you suffer from cluster migraines, it may be helpful to avoid foods containing nitrites as well as medications containing histamine and other ingredients that might dilate blood vessels. You should therefore familiarize yourself with the effects of foods, beverages, and medications that tend to dilate your blood vessels. You'll learn more about this in Chapter 2.

Since a cluster headache often goes into remission for months or years at a time, you should not assume that you have found a cure for the headache when it does not recur for a while. You should continue to practice prevention every day by avoiding any possible food or factor in your environment that might trigger a cluster headache.

Tracking Type M Headaches

Type O headaches are often severe and persistent and are frequently accompanied by other symptoms, such as nausea or visual disturbances. Simple Type M headaches are often due to tightness in the neck and shoulders, triggered by fatigue or stress. While there are many things you can do

1

to help prevent and relieve some types of Type O headaches, such as migraine, you should always be under the care of a physician. When it has been established that your headache is of the Type M variety, the most common type of headache, treatment and prevention will be entirely up to you. Chapter 2 will tell you how to relieve tension headache as well as how to prevent vascular headaches caused by foods and environmental factors.

Headaches that are difficult to diagnose might require the special abilities of a physician who can recognize the symptoms of such problems as glaucoma, mastoiditis, lead poisoning, carbon monoxide inhalation, food allergies, ketosis from rapid weight loss, kidney failure, and other conditions in which headache is only one of many symptoms. There are headache clinics throughout the United States where you can receive special attention for an undiagnosed headache.

How to Determine the Cause of Your Neck, Shoulder, and Arm Pain

Neck, shoulder, or arm pain can occur separately or in combination and may or may not be related to a neck problem. It usually takes a little detective work to determine the source of the pain. With a little instruction, you can become a pretty good medical sleuth. And you can feel confident in offering your services to other members of your family when the need arises.

That Pain in Your Neck

Neck pain is most often musculoskeletal in nature; that is, mechanical or Type M. Neck pain referred from some other portion of the body through connecting nerve fibers is less common but more serious and should be diagnosed without delay. A heart, lung, gall bladder, or blood vessel problem, for example, commonly refers pain to the neck.

Generally, there is one simple way to distinguish Type M from Type O neck pain. If you feel pain in your neck when you move your head or lift your arms, chances are the muscles and joints of the neck are involved. In a simple muscle spasm or "crick," for example, which often occurs on one side of the neck and upper back, rotating the head toward the painful side will usually intensify the pain and restrict movement. When neck pain is relieved by rest or immobility and aggravated by movement, the problem is probably mechanical and not serious. If the pain is constant and is not affected by movement of the neck, however, there may be a possibility that the pain is being referred to the neck from somewhere else.

A Case of Type O Neck Pain

A patient came into my office complaining of a severe neck pain that did not affect movement of his neck and that could not be aggravated by mechanical testing, such as placing pressure on the cervical spine and its supporting muscles. A history of heart trouble prompted referral to a cardiologist who diagnosed pericarditis, an inflammation of the lining surrounding the heart.

For home diagnosis, it's enough to know that *pain not aggravated by movement might be coming from an internal source, while pain relieved by rest and increased by movement is probably mechanical in nature.*

Be on guard, however. Persistent pain that is unrelieved by rest but is aggravated by movement might be indicative of a potentially serious joint problem. Constant, progressively increasing pain that is worse at night but is not aggravated by movement might be an indication of disease inside the bone. If you have a history of any form of cancer, prostate or uterine cancer in particular, you should bring your history as well as your symptoms to the attention of a doctor.

Arm Pain Originating in the Neck

Shoulder and arm pain commonly originates in the neck, even when there is no neck pain. This usually happens when a bony spur, a bulging disc, or some other abnormality in the neck presses on a spinal nerve referring symptoms into a portion of the arm. A "pinched nerve" can often be recognized as a persistent numbness, tingling, or aching that radiates into the shoulder and down the arm. Usually the symptoms will be present only in one portion of the shoulder or arm, often involving two or three fingers. The location of the symptoms will correspond to certain vertebrae or discs in the cervical spine, enabling your doctor to determine exactly where the pain originates. If necessary, he or she may then order an X ray or MRI exam.

Arm Pain Originating in the Shoulder

When you have pain in your upper arm, your shoulder should always be examined, since the shoulder will often radiate symptoms as far down as the elbow.

A Test for Shoulder Trouble

You can test your shoulder joint simply by reaching back in an attempt to scratch your back or by lifting your arm in all directions. If movement is restricted by pain in any direction, you may have a shoulder problem. If movement of the shoulder does not cause pain, the pain in your upper arm may be coming from your neck. When this is the case, arm pain caused by a pinched nerve in your neck can often be relieved by placing your arm over your head. When a patient walks into my office with his forearm resting on top of his head, the diagnosis is almost always cervical nerve root impingement causing shoulder and arm pain.

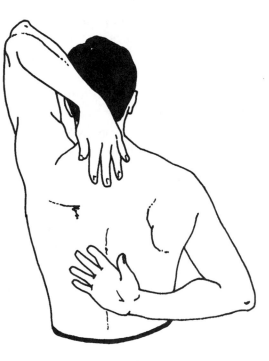

Figure 1-1. Shoulder pain caused by attempting to scratch your back between your shoulder blades may be a sign of a mechanical-type shoulder problem, such as tendonitis, as opposed to referred pain from the cervical spine.

Note: In tendonitis, or inflammation of a tendon near the shoulder socket, pain and restricted movement may occur only when the arm is moved in a certain direction. The direction of movement causing pain—forward, out to the side, or back—will provide a clue as to which tendon is involved. Your doctor might then say that you have a supraspinatus tendonitis, calcific tendonitis, or a rotator cuff problem, which are all tendon problems involving the shoulder socket, as opposed to radiculitis or radiculopathy involving an inflamed or damaged cervical nerve.

When bursitis (inflammation of a lubricating sac) or arthritis (inflammation of joint surfaces) is present in a shoulder socket, movement in all directions may be painful.

Be sure to read Chapter 3 if you have any kind of shoulder pain.

The Mystery of Elbow Pain

A pinched nerve in the neck will sometimes refer pain to the elbow. Such pain will have no effect on movement of the elbow. When pain originates in the elbow itself, however, movement of the elbow will be painful. The pain of elbow tendonitis or tennis elbow, for example, may be increased by gripping objects or by turning doorknobs. The pain of elbow arthritis can be felt simply by bending or twisting the elbow.

Obviously, when pain in the elbow is referred from the neck, you should treat the neck and not the elbow. When you do apply treatment to an elbow, make sure that it's your elbow and not your neck or shoulder that needs treatment.

You'll learn in Chapter 3 how to relieve referred pain in your arm. Chapter 8 will tell you how to use home remedies to relieve arthritis and tendonitis in your elbow.

The Flip Side of Wrist Pain

A nerve will sometimes get pinched between the bones and ligaments on the palm side of the wrist, causing pain, numbness, and weakness in the hand and fingers (carpal tunnel syndrome). Bending the wrist downward forcefully may increase pain and numbness in the fingers by increasing pressure on the impinged nerve (Phalan's sign). Tapping over the damaged nerve on the palm side of the wrist with the fingertips may produce numbness in the fingers, especially in the middle long finger (Tinel's sign). Testing by a neurologist may be needed to confirm such pinching.

Surgery is sometimes performed to relieve the symptoms of carpal tunnel syndrome. You'll learn in Chapter 3 how you might be able to avoid surgery by taking a special vitamin supplement or by wearing a wrist splint.

Note: When a wrist or an elbow swells from inflammation, special blood tests might be needed to diagnose possible rheumatoid or gouty arthritis, both of which must be treated medically.

Arm Symptoms Caused by a Neck Muscle

Occasionally, nerves may be irritated and blood flow restricted by pressure on nerves and blood vessels in the neck having nothing to do with the cervical spine. Such a problem might cause pain, numbness, tingling, and vascular symptoms in the *entire arm and hand*, especially when you are in certain postures. This condition can be caused by an extra rib in the neck or by an abnormal neck (scalenus) muscle. Doctors might call the condition a scalenus anticus syndrome, a thoracic outlet syndrome, or a cervical rib syndrome (if a cervical rib is present).

You can test for this condition in the following manner: Stand erect with your arms hanging close to your sides. Have someone feel the pulse in the wrist of the affected arm. Turn your head to the opposite side and hold it there for several seconds. If your pulse is diminished or obliterated, this means that blood vessels supplying your arm and hand are being compressed in your neck by a rib or a muscle. Compression of brachial nerves in the neck may also cause numbness or tingling in your arm.

Cervical traction, or stretching your neck, will often relieve arm pain caused by nerves pinched in the spinal joints, but such treatment might aggravate the pain of a scalenus anticus or cervical rib problem. Remember that a cervical rib is an *extra* rib, attached to the last (seventh) cervical vertebra in your neck. Its presence sometimes encroaches upon nerves and blood vessels passing above the first thoracic rib, requiring surgical removal in severe cases. A scalenus muscle pressing upon sensitive structures may simply be sectioned or snipped.

Temporary relief for this condition can often be obtained by lifting or supporting the arm above shoulder level to relieve tension on the neck. Changes in work postures or supporting the weight of the arm with a sling might be enough to relieve symptoms.

It's not likely that you'll experience a scalenus anticus or cervical rib syndrome unless you were born with the abnormalities causing these problems. But in order to pinpoint the cause of your arm pain, it would be helpful to distinguish this condition from the typical pinched cervical nerve that would cause pain only in certain portions of your arm or hand, depending upon which vertebra or disc is involved.

How to Analyze Back, Hip, and Leg Pain

Of all the aches and pains we have, back trouble is the most common. Even a fairly minor back problem can be painful and often incapacitating. If you have ever had back pain, you'll want to do all you can to detect, treat, and prevent it with a self-help program.

In distinguishing Type O from Type M back trouble, you should observe pretty much the same basic rules recommended for analyzing neck and arm pains. If pain is relieved by rest and increased by movement or activity, then your trouble is probably mechanical or Type M in nature.

If back pain is persistent, unrelieved by rest, and not aggravated by movement, the pain may have an internal origin. Kidney trouble, for example, is a common cause of Type O backache. If you have a fever that is accompanied by backache and frequent urination, you should have a urinalysis to determine if these symptoms are kidney related.

Note: A urinary stone can cause severe back pain that may radiate into the lower abdomen, groin, and inner thigh on one side, especially when the stone is in the ureter, the tube between the kidney and the bladder. This pain may be accompanied by nausea or vomiting. Unlike severe pain caused by a spinal problem, a urinary stone does not restrict movement, and you may move from one position to another seeking relief from pain; you simply cannot remain still with this condition. A person suffering from severe back pain, on the other hand, will probably lie still because movement causes pain.

If you should be unfortunate enough to suffer from urinary stones, the severe pain may prompt you to visit a hospital emergency room where medication can be administered until you can be examined by a urologist. In a situation like this, you should not call your chiropractor. In my office, if someone calls reporting severe back pain and says that they are walking back and forth or rolling around on the floor, we immediately direct them to a hospital.

A Man's Special Problem

Prostate trouble is a common cause of backache in men. If you are a male over the age of fifty and you have trouble emptying your bladder, requiring you to get up several times a night to dribble a little urine, it's important for you to see a urologist for a prostate examination. A special blood test for prostatic specific antigen (PSA) or acid phosphatase might be done to rule out prostate cancer. Most often, the prostate gland is simply enlarged and sometimes infected. But prostate cancer is so common among elderly men that its presence should always be suspected when there is difficulty emptying the bladder.

Remember that a tumor or a disc protrusion into the spinal canal can cause retention of urine. You'll learn more about this in Chapter 4, but you should always have your physician determine the cause of bladder dysfunction, whether it is the inability to hold urine or the inability to pass urine.

Helping Yourself Find the Right Doctor

Utilizing basic guidelines such as those outlined in this chapter, **Maureen R.** was able to select the type of doctor she needed for her particular problem. "I had a bad backache," she reported, "and it was so bad that I could not sit still. I was about to call my chiropractor when I realized that bending my back did not make the pain worse. So I took my temperature and found that I was running a little fever. It then occurred to me that the frequent urination I was experiencing was not caused by the coffee I was drinking. I went to my family physician who diagnosed a kidney infection."

Like many knowledgeable people, Maureen was able to avoid unnecessary visits to the wrong kinds of doctors by doing a little diagnosis of her own. You can do this too and in the process avoid unnecessary expense and inappropriate treatment.

How the Right Type of Treatment Helped Lester B.

Lester B. also had a backache that was Type O rather than Type M. He did not feel well, his joints ached, and he was having trouble emptying his bladder. He had a constant feeling of urinary urgency. He asked his family physician to refer him to a urologist. A urinalysis and a culture of prostate secretions revealed the presence of white blood cells and pathogenic bacteria, indicating prostate infection as well as bladder infection. With proper treatment, including antibiotics, Lester's back pain and other symptoms disappeared. He was fortunate enough to get treatment that was specific for his back pain.

A knowledge of such simple signs as those observed by Maureen and Lester can be very useful in helping yourself and in selecting a doctor. Of course, a good family physician can help you select a specialist when you need one. But it's always helpful to know enough about your problem so you can avoid the wrong treatment by the wrong kind of doctor.

Since most Type M back problems can be treated at home, you can do much to help yourself if you possess a basic knowledge of how to distinguish Type M from Type O problems.

You Won't Often Need a Specialist

It's rarely necessary to visit a specialist when you experience Type M back pain for the first time. If you do not have a history of back trouble and you hurt your back in some simple activity such as moving furniture, it's not likely that your injury will be serious. Chances are, the pain will disappear after a few weeks of rest. A little physical therapy and a few manipulations by a chiropractor or an osteopath may speed recovery by restoring mobility to stiff muscles and joints if symptoms persist longer than a week. Expensive and possibly harmful examinations such as myelograms (injection of an opaque substance into the spinal canal for imaging purposes) and computerized axial tomography (CAT) scans (computer readings of X-ray impressions that show cross-section pictures of the spine) should not be ordered until time and observation reveal the need for such tests.

In the absence of certain danger signs—such as a history of cancer or major trauma, the presence of fever, age-related osteoporosis, urinary retention or incontinence, pain that is worse at night or at rest, or pain, numbness, or weakness in the legs—*90 percent of people who experience back pain for the first time will recover spontaneously within four weeks.*

If you are feeling fine one day and then hurt your back the next, don't pressure your family physician to send you to a specialist who might send you to a hospital for special testing. Give yourself a little time. Don't panic.

Why Donald S. Didn't Need to See a Doctor

Donald S. was shoveling dirt on his job as a plumber when he heard a "pop" and felt a sharp pain in his lower back. He fell to the ground and was unable to move for a few minutes. When he finally did get back on his feet, Donald asked to be taken to a doctor. "I've never had anything like this," he told his employer. "I might have broken something. I want to see a doctor today."

Donald's problem turned out to be a simple strain. He was doing fine a few weeks later. "I thought I was crippled for life," he confessed with relief.

Most of the time, a back injury like that suffered by Donald, though very painful, will resolve within a week or two, and it's rarely necessary to undergo extensive testing. A visit to your family doctor will usually put your mind at ease. When pain persists or radiates down one of your legs, you should be kept under observation. If symptoms are not relieved in two to

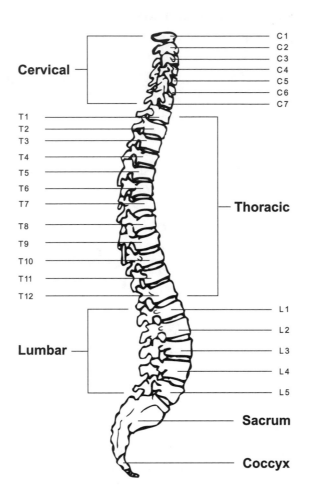

Cervical — C1, C2, C3, C4, C5, C6, C7

Thoracic — T1, T2, T3, T4, T5, T6, T7, T8, T9, T10, T11, T12

Lumbar — L1, L2, L3, L4, L5

Sacrum

Coccyx

Figure 1-2. The spine is a complicated stack of bones held together by ligaments and interlocking joints that are lubricated by synovial sacs and cushioned by intervertebral disc cartilage. There are seven cervical (C), twelve thoracic (T), five lumbar (L), and one sacral (S) vertebrae exiting spinal nerves that supply musculoskeletal structures commonly affected by nerve root irritation. Pain and other symptoms originating in these structures may be difficult to pinpoint but can often be treated successfully with time and self-help. (Figure adapted from Treat Your Back Without Surgery. *© 2002, 1998 by Prizm Development, Inc.)*

four weeks, you may then request examination by a specialist, especially if you are middle-aged or older.

You'll learn more about specialists, what they do, and when to consult them in Chapter 13.

The Many Causes of Back and Leg Pain

Pain radiating down one leg is often caused by a bulging or herniated disc, a bony spur, or some other type M or mechanical problem in the lower back. Leg pain can also be caused by pelvic tumors, prostate disease, bone disease, an abdominal aneurysm, and other Type O problems.

Hip and leg pain not associated with back trouble is sometimes caused by spinal stenosis, or narrowing of the spinal canal and other bony channels that house spinal nerves. When the spinal canal is narrowed, it's called central spinal stenosis. When the openings between the vertebrae are narrowed, it's called lateral spinal stenosis.

With the development of the CAT scan, it's now possible to detect spinal stenosis as well as tumors, herniated discs, and other problems that are difficult to diagnose. Many doctors prefer to use an MRI scan when disc herniation is suspected. Generally, I think of the CAT scan as being best for the study of bones and joints, while MRI is best for the soft tissue studies needed to visualize disc cartilage and nerve tissue. Since MRI involves magnetic resonance Imaging and does not require the use of X-ray radiation, an MRI scan may be the safest as well as the most effective way to locate herniated discs that are pressing against spinal nerves or the spinal cord.

A bone scan will often locate bone disease, tumors, infection, arthritis, or fractures that may not show up on a plain X ray. A radioactive material injected into the bloodstream accumulates in spots where bone is building up or breaking down. These areas show up as "hot spots" when the bones are scanned with a radiation counter.

Type M Back Trouble and How It Can Cause Hip and Leg Pain

In many cases of Type M backache, leg pain will result from irritation or compression of a spinal nerve. When the irritation is originating in the *upper* portion of the lumbar spine (the section of spine just below your ribs), the pain may radiate down the front of the thigh to the knee. Also, trouble in a hip socket can refer pain down the front of the thigh to the knee.

When a spinal nerve is irritated in the *lower* portion of the lumbar spine, most often by a herniated disc, pain may radiate down the back of the thigh to the calf or foot. If this sciatic pain (with numbness and tingling) persists unrelieved, damage to the affected nerve might result in an inability to lift the forepart of your foot, or you might not be able to rise up on your toes. This muscle weakness might cause you to limp or flop your foot when you walk, which is called foot drop.

A Note on the Dangers of X Rays

Since X rays and other diagnostic methods involving radiation can be harmful to your health, they should be used only when absolutely necessary. If you have had recent spinal X rays, try to avoid repeat X rays when you change doctors. X-ray films can be transferred from one doctor to another, and you should always request your X rays when you are referred to another doctor.

When you do have X rays taken of your spine, they should be limited to the painful portion of your back. A few chiropractors, following an unsubstantiated theory, will X-ray your neck to treat your lower back. You can refuse to have such X rays made. Except in rare cases where a scoliosis must be evaluated, full-spine X rays are never necessary. Routine, repeated use of X-ray examinations should be discouraged by the doctor and questioned by the patient. An excessive amount of X rays crashing through your tissue cells, knocking atomic particles out of orbit, can be as harmful as radiation from an atomic bomb. So don't insist on having an X-ray examination if your doctor does not order one. And don't hesitate to refuse unnecessary X-ray duplication.

Remember that MRI does not involve the use of X-ray radiation and is often ordered *after* plain X rays have been made to detect certain mechanical problems.

The Problem of Soft Bones

Anyone with a history of cancer anywhere in the body should be examined periodically when back pain of unknown origin persists. Cancer in the esophagus, lungs, uterus, breast, kidney, thyroid, or prostate gland, for example, can spread to the bones. Blood profiles will often reveal chemical changes that indicate bone or tissue destruction in the body. A high level of calcium and alkaline phosphatase in the blood might be an indication of bone destruction caused by metastatic bone cancer (which has spread from an organ to bone) or by osteogenic sarcoma (a highly malignant tumor that originates in bone), warranting an order for a CAT scan or a bone scan.

Glandular diseases can soften or destroy vertebrae. A tumor in the parathyroid glands in your neck can drain calcium from vertebrae, causing them to collapse or become compressed. A decrease in estrogen levels in calcium-deficient women after menopause may result in osteoporotic crush fractures in thoracic and lumbar vertebrae as a result of hormonal influences draining calcium from bones. Too much adrenal cortical hormone from diseased adrenal glands can also produce bone-softening osteoporosis.

Menopausal women who suffer from arthritis should be cautious about taking cortisone, an adrenal hormone that can contribute to the development of osteoporosis. You'll learn more about this disease in Chapter 4.

Surgery as a Last Resort

We must make a choice between back surgery or a limp when foot drop is imminent. Some of us would prefer surgery in order to relieve damaging pressure on a spinal nerve; others would refuse surgery under any circumstances. Fortunately, spinal or disc surgery is rarely necessary. A physician who keeps a close watch on tendon reflexes will usually advise against surgery if there is no evidence of progressive damage to a compressed nerve.

When disc surgery is necessary to prevent nerve damage or foot drop, neurosurgeons and orthopedic surgeons may now choose from a variety of surgical procedures to remove a herniated disc that is compressing a spinal nerve. A few surgeons remove herniated discs by snipping them out with an aspirating probe (a device that sucks out disc fragments) guided by fluoroscopy or motion X-ray imaging. This procedure is called percutaneous discectomy. Laser energy is also used to burn out herniated disc material. A few doctors still inject an enzyme called chymopapain to dissolve the extruded portion of a herniated disc. New surgical techniques on the horizon will reduce cutting and shorten recovery time.

Remember, however, that disc surgery for back pain without nerve-damage symptoms should be avoided when it is not absolutely necessary. Left alone, your body will eventually dissolve or degenerate a herniated disc, doing its own surgery. Time will often eliminate the need for invasive surgical intervention if progressive nerve damage does not take place. Anything you can do to help yourself avoid surgery may buy the time you need to allow your body to heal itself, relieving back and sciatic leg pain.

According to the guidelines of the Agency for Healthcare Research and Quality cited in the Introduction, "with or without surgery, 80 percent of patients with sciatica recover eventually." The publication also advised that "manipulation [manual movement and stretching of spinal muscles and joints] seems helpful for patients with acute low back problems without

34366000056372

radiculopathy [nerve damage] when used within the first month of symptoms." "Improper treatment," such as prolonged bed rest or unnecessary surgery, results in more disability after treatment than before, the result of "suboptimal care."[2]

If you have been advised to have spinal surgery, get a second opinion from an orthopedist or a neurosurgeon in a teaching hospital where you can also be advised on the latest surgical technique for removing a herniated disc.

Alternatives to Surgery

There are numerous alternatives for avoiding back surgery. Kim T. had suffered from recurring back and leg pain for several months and had been advised to have surgery. Utilizing simple self-help measures such as those outlined throughout this book, from home treatment to changes in posture, Kim eventually recovered from her back and leg pain without surgery. "The time and effort involved in helping myself was certainly worth the effort," she said later. "I did not want a scar on my back if I could avoid it."

There are, of course, cases where surgery is needed to avoid damage to a compressed nerve. An athlete, for example, who is experiencing weakness in flexion or extension (up or down movement) of a foot from a pinched spinal nerve might prefer surgery to a permanent calf and foot weakness that would hinder athletic performance. Most young persons who want to avoid a foot-flopping weakness for cosmetic reasons would prefer surgery as well.

Why Alfred A. Chose Not to Have Back Surgery

Fifty-year-old Alfred A. was told that he would develop a permanent weakness in the muscles of his lower leg if he did not have back surgery. Since Alfred was not a physically active person, he chose the muscle weakness over the surgery. When the pain finally disappeared, the muscles in the affected calf had atrophied (shrunken), and there was a numbness over a portion of his leg and foot. "The limp doesn't bother me a bit," he insisted. "Besides, I'm past the age where I'm concerned about how I look." You might feel differently, however, and prefer the scar and the risk of surgery to a physical impairment, however minor.

When your doctor recommends surgery, always ask what the alternatives are so that you can weigh the consequences of having the surgery or refusing the surgery. The choice is always yours. If your doctor refuses to discuss your problem with you, go to another doctor. Spinal surgery is no small matter when it is performed on *you*, and you are entitled to answers for any question you have.

Above all, do all you can to relieve symptoms and avoid surgery. Use of many of the self-help measures described in this book will help you avoid surgery as well as *prevent* the development of serious back trouble. So, even if your back trouble is not yet a major problem, you can do a lot to make sure that it does not become one.

Watch for Circulatory Symptoms!

Most of the time pain in the leg will originate in the lower spine where a spinal nerve is being compressed or irritated. You must always be on the lookout for leg pain caused by a circulatory problem, however, especially if you are past middle age. *Blockage or obstruction of an artery in the leg can be much more serious than a pinched nerve.* In the case of a blood clot or a clogged artery, serious damage can occur in a short period of time. Treatment must be given immediately, especially if you are elderly or have diabetes.

A pinched nerve, while painful, does not present an immediate threat. The worst that can happen is muscle weakness and loss of sensation in only a portion of the affected leg. A clogged artery, however, can result in loss of a leg or a foot.

Usually, the pain resulting from an obstructed artery is so severe that the victim will seek medical care. I have known of cases, however, where the pain of a circulatory obstruction was confused with the pain of a pinched nerve, allowing the development of gangrene in a foot and its toes.

There are some basic guidelines that you can follow in distinguishing a clogged artery from a pinched nerve.

Leg pain caused by a pinched nerve is often associated with numbness and tingling and may be located in an isolated portion of the leg, ankle, or foot. Such pain may be accompanied by back trouble and appear to radiate from the hip to the leg. It is often described as a "deep bone pain" or a cramping pain that is aggravated by standing and relieved by lying down.

In the case of a blood clot or a clogged artery, a severe leg pain may appear suddenly without warning and without any associated back trouble. Severe, unrelenting pain involving the entire leg and foot, unaffected by rest or movement, may be accompanied by cold, discoloration, and loss of ankle pulse. Since nicotine can reduce circulation by constricting blood vessels, you should quit smoking at the first sign of a circulatory problem. Buerger's disease, characterized by inflammation and clogging of arteries in the legs, occurs predominantly in twenty- to forty-year-old men who smoke. Another reason to quit smoking!

Intermittent Claudication: The Walking Pain

Leg pain caused by hardened arteries (intermittent claudication) occurs primarily while walking. If your calves consistently cramp after walking a block or two and are immediately relieved by rest, you may assume that poor blood flow in hard, narrow arteries is keeping your leg muscles from receiving adequate oxygen. The aching, cramping pain of vascular intermittent claudication can occur in the foot, thigh, hip, and buttocks, as well as in the calf. Most of the time, however, symptoms will occur only in the calf.

(Neurogenic claudication, or pain in both legs caused by central spinal stenosis or pressure inside the spinal canal, may occur when standing at rest rather than when walking. Pain is likely to be aggravated by coughing and sneezing. The ankle pulse will be normal. Spinal stenosis can be caused by congenital (existing at birth) narrowing of the spinal canal or by diseases that thicken bones and ligaments, as in Paget's disease. Aging sometimes thickens a spinal ligament called the *ligamentum flavum,* which bulges into the spinal canal.)

Unlike the walking pain caused by hardened arteries, which is relieved by rest, the pain of a blood clot in a major leg artery will persist during rest. So it's not likely that you will confuse the symptoms of a clot-obstructed artery with the intermittent claudication caused by hardened arteries. Nor is it likely that you will confuse either of these problems with the numbness and tingling of a pinched nerve that is associated with back trouble. You can help your doctor diagnose your problem by describing your symptoms as clearly as you can.

Once it has been established that your leg pain is being caused by hardened arteries, you should walk as much as you can to improve circulation in your legs. Walk until the pain begins, then stop and rest until the pain subsides, then begin walking again. Going on a low-fat diet (see Chapter 6) and supplementing your diet with a few hundred units of vitamin E might help keep your arteries open.

Ten Tests for Type M Back Pain

Here are ten simple tests you can do safely at home to determine if your low-back pain is mechanical in nature. Try them all, but discontinue a test if it begins to cause back pain.

1. **The standing bend test:** Stand erect and bend from side to side, forward, and backward. If you feel pain or obvious discomfort during any of these movements, it's likely that you have a low-back problem that might involve muscles or joints. Be sure to keep your legs straight while bending so that movement takes place in your spine and not just in your hips and knees, but *do not try to touch your toes.*

    If you have a back problem, you might notice that you tend to keep your back flat while bending forward, bending at the hips in order to reduce movement in your lower back.

2. **The spinal percussion test:** Have someone lightly jar the painful area of your spine with a closed fist. Instruct the examiner to straddle the spinous processes (the bony projections in the middle of your back) with the first two fingers of one hand and then lightly pound on the fingers with the bottom of a closed fist to help you jar and locate sensitive structures.

    If there is a spinal problem severe enough to cause swelling around joints and ligaments, or if there is bone disease or a disc herniation, you can locate the exact level of the problem by eliciting pain with percussion.

3. **The heel-drop test:** Rise up on your toes and drop your full weight on your heels. If you feel pain in your back when your heels hit the floor, you have another confirmation that you might have trouble involving your vertebrae. The jar of your heels striking the floor simply bangs sensitive joints together.

4. **The toe-walk test:** Walk across the floor on your toes. If you cannot support your weight on the toes of one foot or the other, you might have a weak calf muscle from nerve damage caused by a herniated disc in your lower spine, especially if you have been having leg pain.

Weakness in one of your thighs while squatting can indicate disc herniation in the *upper* portion of your lumbar spine.

You might be able to detect muscle atrophy or shrinkage in the affected leg or thigh by measuring both legs with a tape. A difference greater than a quarter of an inch might be significant. Your doctor will be able to confirm nerve damage by checking the tendon reflexes in your ankles or your knees.

5. **The heel-walk test:** Try walking on your heels. If you cannot hold the forepart of one or both feet off the floor while heel walking, you might be developing "foot drop," a weakness caused by damage to a spinal nerve that reaches from your lower lumbar spine to a shin muscle.

   Rub the skin over the involved shin and see if it feels numb. If it does, tell your doctor about it when you describe the weakness in your foot.

6. **The straight-leg-raise test:** Lie flat on your back. Raise one leg straight up, as high as you can. If you feel pain in your back, hip, and leg while lifting your leg 30 to 70 degrees, you might have nerve root impingement in your lower spine (Lasègue's sign). Test and compare both legs. The affected leg cannot be raised as high (because of pain) as the unaffected leg.

   If raising the unaffected leg causes pain on the opposite side, this "crossover sign" may be an indication of massive disc herni-

Figure 1-3. "Pinched nerve" symptoms commonly originate in the lower back, most often as a result of disc herniation, causing pain, numbness, and other symptoms to radiate down the leg. Symptoms aggravated by straight-leg raising, which stretches the sciatic nerve, may be indicative of nerve root entrapment and should be brought to the attention of a physician.

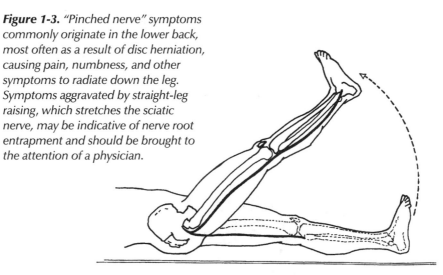

ation. This most commonly occurs in the last two discs of the spine—at the L4 or the L5 level (see illustration on page 18).

If you simply have tight hamstrings, you won't be able to raise either leg very high—not because of pain but because of stiffness or pulling behind your knees. If pain occurs on one side on the back of the pelvis, you might have a sacroiliac problem, indicating strain or disease in the joint between the sacrum and the pelvis.

Note: This test is best performed with someone helping you raise the straight leg. When the leg is raised to the point of pain, forced flexion of the foot (moving the forepart of the foot toward of the shin) by the helper will increase pain in the hip and behind the knee if there is impingement of a spinal nerve.

7. **The leg-hold test:** Extend and lift both legs several inches off the floor (while lying on your back) and hold them there for a few seconds. If you feel pain in the middle of your lower back, your lower spine may have been affected by disease or injury or you may have a bulging disc.

   In acute low-back conditions, the pull of your psoas, or hip-flexor muscles, on your lumbar vertebrae during a double-leg lift might trigger a sharp low-back pain if you have a bulging disc or swelling around the joints in the lower lumbar area.

8. **The Figure-4 hip test:** While lying flat on your back, place the ankle of one foot on the knee of the opposite leg to form the figure 4. Relax and let the knee of the bent leg sag. If pain

Figure 1-4. "Figure-4" testing is positive for a hip socket problem when pain or locking prevents lowering of the knee from the position shown in this illustration.

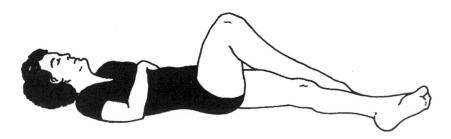

occurs in the groin area of the bent leg, you might have a hip-socket problem that could cause pain to radiate down the front of your thigh to your knee. It might also cause pain on one side of the back of your pelvis if you have a sacroiliac problem.

Test both hips equally. The knee on the side of the bad hip might "hang up" as a result of binding in a bad hip socket so that it does not drop as low as the knee on the unaffected side.

9. **The femoral stretch test:** Lie face down and bend one leg, lifting the heel toward your buttocks. If pain occurs in your back and the front of the thigh of the flexed leg, you might have nerve-root impingement in the upper portion of your lumbar spine.

    If you have pain radiating down the front of your thigh to your knee, try both the figure-4 and the femoral stretch test to determine if the pain is coming from your back or from your hip.

10. **The cough test:** If you feel back pain when you cough, sneeze, or turn over in bed, or while getting up from a sitting position, getting in and out of your car, or while leaning over to wash your face, you obviously have a low-back problem that is probably mechanical or Type M.

    Simply tilting your head down to get in and out of your car will aggravate acute mechanical-type low-back pain.

Solutions for Your Problems

Now that you have some idea of how to determine what is causing your head, neck, arm, back, or leg problem, you probably want to help relieve your aches and pains.

You'll find plenty of home remedies for Type M back trouble and all its associated problems—from arthritis to muscle spasm—in the remaining chapters of this book. Just turn to the chapter that interests you most. However, be sure to read all the other chapters for the information you need to prevent other types of aches and pains.

SUMMARY

1. Self-help in the care of head, neck, arm, back, and leg pain is effective primarily in the care of mechanical or Type M conditions involving muscles, joints, and ligaments.

2. When pain persists or is accompanied by fever and other symptoms, ask your doctor to examine you to determine if an organic or Type O problem involving disease or infection exists.

3. About 90 percent of all headaches are of the tension and migraine variety and can be relieved at home, but you should always be alert to unusual symptoms indicating more serious forms of headaches.

4. A neck problem often results in radiation of pain into the shoulder, arm, and hand.

5. Neck, shoulder, and arm pain not relieved by rest and not increased by movement might be referred pain from a pinched nerve or a diseased organ.

6. A shoulder problem, indicated by pain on movement of the shoulder, will often refer pain into the upper arm.

7. Low-back trouble is the most common of the Type M problems and is often responsible for pain referred into the hip, thigh, and leg.

8. A hip problem, indicated by testing of the hip socket, can refer pain down the front of the thigh to the knee.

9. The self-testing methods described in this book can help you and your doctor determine whether your aches and pains are mechanical or organic in nature.

10. Once it has been determined that you are suffering from a mechanical or Type M problem, you can help yourself with a variety of home remedies—and there is much you can do to prevent a recurrence of symptoms.

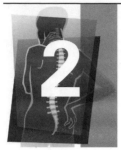

Headache: Home Treatment and Prevention

Headache is nearly as common as backache. Ninety percent of the population experiences occasional headache, which is the tension or muscle contraction variety 75 to 80 percent of the time. Since common tension headaches are most often the result of simple muscle tension around the neck and shoulders, there is a lot you can do at home to relieve most headaches.

While home remedies are safe and can be used by anyone, they should be appropriately applied. It's therefore important to remember what was discussed in Chapter 1 about how to recognize signs of brain tumors and other serious causes of Type O head pain.

Fortunately, though, headaches are rarely serious. Migraine headache, while not life-threatening, can cause such severe symptoms that they should always be investigated to rule out organic disease. Any headache that is accompanied by visual disturbances, fever, vomiting, diarrhea, and other symptoms of illness warrants medical attention.

Generally, and luckily for us, it's not too difficult to distinguish simple migraine headache from tension headache. Migraine headache occurs only occasionally, never daily, and most often in females. They are usually associated with an aura (a premonitory feeling or sensation) that warns you of an impending "sick headache," as they are sometimes called. Cluster headache occurs most often in males and is a less common but more severe form of migrainous pain that is accompanied by watering of the eye and blockage of the nostril on the affected side. This type of headache can occur daily for weeks at a time and then disappear for months. Simple headache that comes and goes on a daily basis is almost always the result of fatigue or tension. Anything that causes a "pain in the neck" can trigger a tension headache.

Self-Help with Home Remedies

If you feel that you have the type of headache that might benefit from any of the variety of home remedies described in this chapter, you should certainly try them. Be sure to read the entire chapter, however; you might recognize a cause for your headache in such simple things as eating a hot dog or drinking a glass of wine.

How John T. Learned to Prevent Vascular Headaches by Cutting Out Certain Foods

John T. experienced a throbbing headache almost every afternoon on his job as a steelworker. Since medical checkups never revealed a cause for his headaches, he assumed that his pain was caused by stress. I questioned John about his eating habits and learned that his lunch usually consisted of hot dogs or lunchmeats.

"You might be having a vascular headache triggered by a food additive," I told John. "Quit eating wieners and lunchmeats that are preserved with sodium nitrite and see how you get along." When John cut out these food items, his headaches disappeared.

If you are a victim of chronic headaches you, too, may be suffering from reactions caused by eating such things as nitrite-preserved meats, salty snacks, or Chinese food containing monosodium glutamate (MSG). Missing a meal, smoking cigarettes, drinking coffee, and many other things we all do every day can trigger a headache in susceptible persons. Wine, chocolate, and cheese are often blamed for migraine or vascular headaches. You'll learn how this happens when you read the rest of this chapter.

In some cases, headaches can be prevented simply by eliminating an obvious cause. When the cause is not known, you may try using basic home remedies to see if they help. Even if you do not find a way to prevent your headache, you may be able to do something to relieve your symptoms.

How Ernestine R. Relieved Chronic Headaches with Self-Care

Ernestine R. had been experiencing chronic, recurring headache for years. "I have this dull, throbbing headache," she explained, "and it hurts from the back of my head to my eyebrows. Sometimes it's so bad that the top of my head and the muscles in my neck are sore to touch. I've been to many doctors, and none of them can find anything wrong. I usually end up with a prescription for muscle relaxants, painkillers, or tranquilizers. I've spent a fortune on doctors and medicines, but I keep having headaches. Lately, I've been having stomach trouble and a skin rash that my doctor says might be caused by the medicine I'm taking. What am I going to do?"

Since all of Ernestine's medical tests were consistently negative, and since she was a high-strung person who would probably have recurring tension-type headaches, I advised her to quit taking medication and to try home remedies on a daily basis. I also advised her to exercise regularly, eat properly, and get adequate rest.

Along with a change in lifestyle, Ernestine massaged the back of her neck under a hot shower each night and then had her husband stretch her neck a little. The results were dramatic.

"I can't believe that a few simple treatments at home could do so much good," Ernestine reported incredulously. "My headaches have nearly disappeared. Now, when I do have a headache, I can ease it with moist heat and a little neck stretching. I'm feeling so much better that my husband and I are going bowling two nights a week. We're also visiting more frequently in our bedroom!"

Simple Techniques to Relieve Tension Headaches

As you know by now, most tension headaches are caused by tightness in the muscles and joints of the neck. The accumulated lactic acid and other waste products resulting from unrelieved muscle tension irritate nerves and inflame muscles, triggering a headache that usually begins at the back of the head and neck, spreading up over the scalp to the forehead. You can often feel the grip of tight scalp muscles like a band around your head. Arthritis and disc degeneration in the cervical spine can also cause tension-type headaches by tightening neck muscles to protect sensitive joints. Anything you can do to break this vicious cycle would be a blessing.

First, Try Moist Heat

The simplest, most effective way to relax tense muscles is to apply moist heat directly to the involved muscles. Moist heat, whether applied by a showerhead or a hot pack, dilates blood vessels and warms and relaxes muscles, flushing out waste products.

The easiest way to do this is to stand under a hot shower and let the water run over the back of your neck and shoulders. If you do not have a good showerhead that releases a broad, heavy spray of water, go out and buy one. There are many good "shower massagers" on the market. A really good showerhead costs considerably more than the small, conventional showerheads, but they are worth the price for their therapeutic effect.

If moist heat does not seem to help and you feel that your neck muscles are inflamed and in spasm, try a cold pack. Cold eases pain by numbing nerve endings. It may also reduce muscle spasm by decreasing metabolic activity in the spastic muscles. Use whichever feels best to you, but try moist heat first. You can buy a special cervical pack that can be heated in a microwave oven or cooled in a freezer. Drape this pack, hot or cold, over the back of your neck and go about your business.

The cervical pack is a godsend for many of us who are too busy to lie down with a hot pack or a cold pack. I have prescribed this pack for secretaries and clerks as well as for overworked housewives.

You'll find instructions later in this chapter on how to make a simple cold pack on your own.

Special Moist Heat Rolls

A moist heat application applied to the neck with a hot compress is probably the best way to stimulate blood flow in tight neck muscles, since the effect is more localized. You may simply wring out towels in hot water and drape them over the back of your neck, or you can make a special *fomentation roll.*

Roll up a hot, wet cotton towel in dry flannel to make a cervical fomentation. The cotton towel will hold moisture while the flannel will hold in the heat. Flannel blankets, which are about half wool and half cotton, will hold both heat and moisture and can be used to wrap around cotton towels.

Wrap the fomentation around your neck, or drape it over the back of your neck, and leave it there until the fomentation cools. Repeat the application two or three times—or until your neck feels relaxed.

A Special Neck Massage Technique

After your neck muscles have been relaxed by moist heat applications, or your pain has been relieved by a cold pack, you can use a special massage technique to break down tissue deposits so that they can be flushed out by the flow of blood. The secret of this technique is that special attention is given to the muscle attachments at the top of the neck near the base of the skull. In addition to the effects of kneading, the firm pressure used in the application of this massage will stimulate your body's production of endorphin, a natural painkiller.

Demonstrate the following massage technique on a friend or mate and then have him or her apply the treatment to your neck.

Have your partner sit on a chair or a stool. If you are right-handed, place the palm of your left hand on your partner's forehead. Instruct your partner to tilt his head forward and relax his neck muscles so that your hand is supporting his head. Encircle the back of your partner's neck at the base of his skull with the thumb and forefinger of your right hand. Exert a little pressure and move your massaging hand up and down in a short circular motion so that the skin moves over the muscles without surface friction. A few seconds of firm kneading in this manner will press out waste products and make room for a cleansing flow of blood.

How Calvin T. Uses Massage to Relieve Tension Headaches

Calvin T., a professional football player, relieves his pregame nervous tension headaches by having the team trainer use this special massage technique on him before a game. "I showed the technique to the trainer and then had him use it on me," he explained. "It always relieves my headache, and I perform much better throughout the game."

For additional home massage, try this: Put a little cream or oil on the *back* of your neck and across the top of your shoulders. Reach across with your right arm and use your fingertips to rub from the tip of your shoulder to the bottom of your neck and then from the top of your neck to the bottom of your neck on the left side. Repeat several times. Then use your left hand to massage your shoulder and neck muscles in the same manner on the right side.

Remove the lubricant by rubbing with a dry towel or with alcohol and a paper towel. Then place both hands on the back of your neck at the base of your skull. Tilt your head forward and press forward and up to stretch the muscles on the back of your neck. You can do this simple neck-stretching exercise anywhere.

A Bedroom Neck-Stretching Technique

If your headache does not respond to these remedies, another neck-stretching exercise performed by a partner might do the trick.

Lie on your back with your head at the foot of the bed. Instruct your partner to grip your neck at the base of your skull. Then have your partner lift your head a little and pull slowly and smoothly until your neck is comfortably stretched as far as it will go. Easy does it! Keep your neck muscles relaxed while the stretch is being applied. The pull should be released and repeated two or three times. Stop the stretching if you experience any pain, discomfort, or dizziness.

Don't be alarmed if your neck clicks or pops while it is being stretched. The popping you hear—or feel—is merely a sudden and harmless separation of joint surfaces, like the cracking of a knuckle.

Neck cracking, a cervical manipulation, or "adjustment," of the vertebrae in the cervical spine, performed by a chiropractor or an osteopath, is often effective in the treatment of tension headache. Because of the danger of injury to the arteries in your neck, however, you should not receive such treatment if you are taking blood thinners or if a preliminary examination by your doctor reveals clogging (noise) in your carotid arteries or if dizziness occurs when you turn your head from side to side. (Remember that an inner ear problem can also cause dizziness when you tilt your head.) When in doubt, it's always best to first try moist heat, massage, and gentle neck stretching at home to see if that will help before trying cervical manipulation. Cervical manipulation is explained in greater detail in Chapter 3.

Solo Neck Stretching with a Head Harness

Neck traction with a head harness with weights ranging from 5 to 15 pounds for a few minutes at a time will often prevent or relieve tension headache.

If the simple neck-stretching techniques described in this chapter do not work for you, try the head harness traction described in Chapter 3. Neck stretching with a head harness and a pulley will enable you to select the amount of pull that feels best to you. Best of all, you can carry your head harness around with you, on the job or when you travel, so that you can use it when you need it—all by yourself and for as long as you like. You can purchase a cervical traction apparatus, with instructions for its use, without a prescription in almost any drugstore.

What Walter, Alice, and Arthur Do to Relieve
Their Headaches

Walter D., a forty-four-year-old traveling salesman, frequently suffers from neck pain and tension headache after long hours of driving night and day on busy highways. After a long drive he rigs up his neck traction and stretches his neck for ten or fifteen minutes with a 15-pound sandbag. "The neck stretching always relieves my headache," he says. "I don't know how I would get by without it."

Alice T. would develop a tension headache within minutes after a stressful meeting with her in-laws. "My in-laws are a pain in the neck," she complained. "I can always expect a headache when they visit my home. Fortunately, I have learned how to lie down and relax my muscles so totally that I can usually ease my headache by thinking it away."

You might be able to "think away" your headaches, too, if you'll spend a little time learning how to relax your muscles with your mind. I'll tell you how later in this chapter.

Sometimes, a number of factors will combine to trigger a severe headache. Arthur T., for example, often experienced a tension headache at the end of the day, but could usually relieve his symptoms with a little rest and neck massage. If he wasn't careful to eat properly, get adequate rest, and avoid stress, however, he was sure to get a migraine-type headache.

How to Use Rest and Relaxation to Relieve
Tension Headaches

Rest, sleep, and relaxation of muscles are all helpful in relieving most types of headaches, especially tension headache. Simply getting a good night's sleep will often provide the rest and relaxation you need. During the day, however, when you are not able to unload your responsibilities and go to bed, you might be able to relieve tension by taking a few minutes to concentrate on relaxing your muscles. With practice, you should be able to relax at will. You can learn to do this by lying down and progressively, systematically contracting and relaxing your muscles, one set at a time, concentrating on relaxing until you are as limp as a rag doll. This method of inducing relaxation, known as the Jacobson technique, was first developed in 1929 and has been a popular medical prescription ever since. You begin by contracting and relaxing the muscles of your feet, then your calves, then your thighs, and so on, working your way from your feet to your scalp until each set of muscles is relaxed.

Such relaxation techniques are actually a form of do-it-yourself biofeedback. After a while, you'll be able to tell whether you are relaxed or tense simply by the way your body feels.

Deep breathing also induces relaxation by blowing off carbon dioxide, increasing blood flow to the brain, and slowing down the sympathetic nervous system. Lie down and breathe deeply, first deep into your abdomen and then high up into your chest. Stop when you begin to feel dizzy from hyperventilation. You can combine deep breathing and progressive muscle relaxation techniques to produce relaxation with a sense of euphoria.

If all else fails, soaking in a tub of warm water at the end of the day is a sure way to induce relaxation of muscles.

Note: Lying down will relieve most headaches caused by tension in muscles around the neck and shoulders. Persons suffering from headache caused by histamine or cluster headache, however, might have to remain in an upright or inclined position to avoid an increase in pressure in swollen, sensitive blood vessels around the head. A warm glass of milk, a good source of the amino acid tryptophan, may help induce sleep. Serotonin, a chemical that transmits messages in the brain and promotes relaxation, is synthesized from tryptophan, which is supplied by turkey and some other fresh, natural foods.

Sufferers of common migraine report that lying down and resting in a darkened room often helps relieve symptoms, while persons suffering from more severe classic migraine might have to keep their head elevated to ease throbbing pain. Go by the way you feel. You can learn from experience which position is best for you.

How to Relieve Head Pain with an Ice Pack

When throbbing head pain persists despite everything you do to relieve it, an ice pack might help. Since dilated scalp and temporal blood vessels are often present in sick or vascular-type headaches, a cold pack placed over the forehead, the temples, or the neck for about twenty minutes will sometimes relieve pain by constricting blood vessels and reducing blood flow.

You can make an ice pack by placing ice cubes and a little water in a Ziploc bag, squeezing out the air before zipping the bag shut, and wrapping it in a dry hand towel.

A hot footbath combined with a cold pack on the head or neck might relieve a vascular-type headache by drawing blood to the feet from swollen blood vessels in the face, head, and neck.

Blood vessels around the brain and in the scalp may dilate in a vascular headache, and some headache victims report that wrapping a tight bandage around the head relieves head pain by compressing blood vessels in the scalp.

Coffee and Cigarettes Constrict Blood Vessels

The caffeine in a cup of brewed coffee is a potent vasoconstrictor. A cup of strong coffee might occasionally be more effective than an ice pack in relieving the throbbing pain of a vascular headache. This is why some headache medications often contain caffeine along with aspirin or acetaminophen. More than two cups of coffee might trigger headache in susceptible persons, however, by stimulating the adrenal glands to cause hypoglycemia, a debilitating drop in blood sugar.

If you do drink coffee, be careful not to develop a caffeine habit. Drink in moderation. Excessive consumption of coffee can result in headaches caused by caffeine withdrawal. If you're accustomed to drinking large amounts of coffee every day, blood vessels that are conditioned by vasoconstricting caffeine might react by *dilating* when you do not meet your usual coffee intake.

Another warning about coffee: It's well known that the caffeine in coffee is a nervous system stimulant that, when consumed in the evening, will prevent some persons from sleeping. Since rest and sleep are important in recovering from headache, you should not drink coffee late in the day when you feel that you need a good night's sleep. In the evening, a warm bath and a relaxing massage, or even an ounce or two of alcohol, may be more appropriate than a cup of coffee.

The nicotine in tobacco products is also a vasoconstrictor that can produce a rebound vascular headache when a smoker is deprived of nicotine. If you smoke cigarettes, quit! In addition to addictive headache, smoking has been directly linked to cancer, heart disease, stroke, and other fatal illnesses.

Alcohol and Headache

While caffeine in coffee constricts blood vessels and stimulates nerves, alcohol dilates blood vessels and relaxes muscles. Excessive consumption of alcohol, however, can cause a throbbing headache by overly dilating blood vessels or by triggering hypoglycemia. The hangover headache is a familiar price that must be paid the day after overindulgence in alcoholic drinks. Obviously, you should not drink alcohol when you have a vascular headache.

Alcohol, like caffeine, tends to destroy B vitamins in your body, contributing to the development of headache. If you drink alcohol or smoke cigarettes and you have headaches, take a vitamin B complex supplement along with a little extra vitamin C.

Headache-Causing Amines in Wine and Cheese

Chemical compounds called amines, commonly found in wine and cheese, can be a cause of headache. Although amines are essential for the function of your brain and your blood vessels, too much of certain amines can lead to the vascular reaction that causes migraine. Red wine, brandy, and sherry are high in the amines known to cause headache. So are cheddar, stilton, and blue cheese, which are rich in tyramine, the amine that most commonly triggers headaches.

If you tend to suffer from headache after drinking wine, try drinking white wine rather than red. It might also be a good idea to avoid cheese snacks while drinking wine. Remember, however, that too much wine or alcohol of any kind can dilate blood vessels and cause a vascular headache.

Hot Dog Headaches

Headaches are sometimes caused by food. One type of food-related headache is caused by a food allergy, for example to wheat products, citrus fruits, eggs, dairy products, and seafoods. Fortunately, headaches caused by food allergies are not common.

Processed foods can also cause headache. Artificial ingredients in lunchmeats, for example, include a sodium nitrite preservative, a potent vasodilator that can trigger a vascular headache called "hot dog headache" in susceptible persons. If you experience a throbbing headache with flushing and redness of your face a half hour or so after eating foods containing sodium nitrite, you might be subject to such headaches.

Not everyone is sensitive to the effect of sodium nitrite. People who suffer from migraine headache, however, are likely to be sensitive to any nitrite additive. If you are a headache sufferer, try to avoid preserved meats, such as hot dogs, bacon, ham, salami, sausage, and bologna. Select fresh meats whenever possible.

Nitrites Can Cause Cancer!

Whether you suffer from headaches or not, you should be cautious about consuming foods that contain sodium nitrite. This additive is a known carcinogen that has been linked to cancer in humans.

When you eat meats that have been preserved with sodium nitrite, take vitamin C as soon as possible. There is some evidence to indicate that vitamin C taken with meals may block the conversion of nitrites to cancer-causing nitrosamines in your stomach. If you don't have vitamin C, eat an orange. When you pack a lunch that contains preserved meats, always include an orange.

MSG's Connection to Headaches and Other Unpleasant Vascular Symptoms

Many years ago, a number of people reported that they experienced headache, dizziness, flushing, tingling, and other symptoms after eating in Chinese restaurants. The symptoms were labeled "Chinese restaurant syndrome" and were found to be caused by food heavily seasoned with monosodium glutamate (MSG). Glutamate, an amino acid, is present in most protein foods and gives the foods flavor. When glutamate is isolated and combined with sodium and water, it forms a flavor-enhancing sodium salt of glutamate. Since MSG contains only one-third the amount of sodium as table salt, it is often substituted for salt in a low-sodium diet.

It is the general consensus of the scientific community that use of MSG as an additive to enhance the flavor of foods is safe for the general population, and scientific studies have failed to link MSG to Chinese restaurant syndrome. Anecdotal reports, however, suggest that a small percentage of the population might be sensitive or allergic to MSG.

If you feel that you might be sensitive to MSG, as indicated by flushing and other symptoms, don't add it to your foods. Also, avoid processed snacks flavored with MSG. Since soy sauce and Chinese foods may contain large amounts of MSG, you may have to avoid such foods or at least ask the cook to leave out the additive. Take a look in your kitchen cabinet to see if you are using any flavor enhancers containing MSG. Check the labels on canned and processed foods, such as soup or chips. If you are not a headache victim, don't worry about MSG.

Some steak houses also season with MSG. If you have a headache or a rapid pulse after eating a steak in a restaurant, ask if it uses flavor enhancers.

Too Much Salt Can Cause Headaches

Simply eating heavily salted foods, such as pretzels and potato chips, can trigger headache in susceptible persons.

Too much sodium in any form, especially in such combinations as sodium nitrite and monosodium glutamate, can cause headache. Sodium can also have a harmful effect on your heart and blood vessels. Try to avoid processed foods that contain salt and sodium additives that might harden your arteries and raise your blood pressure. You can get all the sodium you need from fresh, natural foods.

An Elimination Diet for Cluster and Migraine Headaches

Whenever you suspect that a certain food or drink is causing your headache, eliminate that food from your diet for a month and see what happens. Remember that headache resulting from some foods, such as salty nuts, might occur twenty-four hours after their consumption. So it's often difficult to pin down the offending food in one day of observation.

When you experience a headache, make a list of everything you've eaten over the past twenty-four hours to see if you have eaten any of the foods known to cause headache. It might be a good idea to keep a diary of what you eat over a period of a month or so, correlating your eating habits with the appearance of your headaches. Make sure, however, that you continue to eat a variety of foods and maintain a balanced diet.

A Monthly Elimination Diet

If it becomes apparent that certain types of foods are associated with the onset of your headaches, you can try an extended elimination diet. With this method, you eliminate one or two suspected foods from your diet for a month. If headache does not recur during that month, then you might have eliminated the offending food. If headache does occur, put the innocent food back into your diet and eliminate some other suspected food for a month. You can continue this process until you are able to go without a headache for several weeks, indicating that you have eliminated the right food.

Remember that it might be necessary to eliminate, in groups, all foods containing salt, nitrites, monosodium glutamate, and other suspected additives, as well as tyramine-rich foods and beverages. The amines in cheese or chocolate, for example, might continue to cause headache while you are eliminating amine-rich red wine from your diet.

If foods that are not essential to a balanced diet are suspect, they can be eliminated from the diet and then be reintroduced one by one until development of a headache reveals which is the offending food.

Obviously, it will take considerable time, thought, and experimentation to test suspected foods in an elimination diet. It could be worth the effort, however, if the cause of your headache is unknown and you are being forced to take medication to relieve your symptoms.

Environmental Causes of Headaches

Remember that there are many factors other than food that can trigger a headache. Chemical fumes, noise, bright lights, smells, and weather changes, for example, are known trigger factors. Try to avoid exposure to the fumes of paint, unvented heaters, insecticides, aerosol sprays, and other chemicals. Some modern insulation and building materials have been found to contain formaldehyde and other chemicals that might contaminate the air in your home.

Make sure that you get plenty of fresh air when you sleep. Unvented heaters in a tightly sealed room can deprive you of adequate oxygen, forcing carbon dioxide to replace the oxygen in your blood. Burning wood in an open hearth may deplete your home of oxygen, both by combustion and by drawing air up through the chimney. It therefore might not be a good idea to sleep in a room with a burning fireplace.

Stress in your environment can tighten neck muscles enough to cause a tension headache. Extreme, unrelieved stress can produce enough adrenalin to trigger a migraine-type headache.

Exercise as a Treatment for Headaches

Exercise is effective in the treatment and prevention of headaches in a couple of ways. First of all, exercise helps burn off the excess adrenalin produced by the stress of a hard day. It also relaxes tight neck muscles by interrupting the mental processes that are keeping the muscles tight. And probably the most important benefit of all, exercise strengthens the muscles around the neck and shoulders so that they do not fatigue so easily. Almost any kind of exercise will relieve tension and stimulate the production of pain-killing endorphins. But you might need special exercises to strengthen the muscles that support your head, neck, and shoulders.

Two Special Resistive Exercises

Once muscles have been strengthened by regular exercise, they are better able to withstand normal, everyday stress. It's important, however, to make sure that the exercise you do strengthens the muscles above and beyond the strength needed to perform daily tasks. This will provide the reserve strength your muscles need to get you through the day without fatigue or exhaustion. Simple resistive exercise with barbells and dumbbells, which require your muscles to work against controlled resistance, may be the best way to accomplish this.

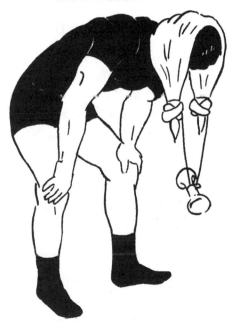

Here are two special resistive exercises that you should include in your training program if you suffer from tension headache caused by weak neck and shoulder muscles that fatigue easily:

1. **Shoulder shrug:** Stand erect with a weight in each hand and shrug your shoulders up and down. Just let the weight hang at arm's length while you lift your shoulders

Figure 2-1. *Neck lifts: This simple resistive neck exercise will strengthen neck muscles on the back of the neck as well as help maintain a normal cervical curve.*

up toward your ears. Shrug your shoulders fifteen times or more while holding 10 pounds or more in each hand. Gradually increase the amount of weight you use as you grow stronger.

2. **Neck lifts:** Cut a strip of sheet or bed spread about 5 feet long and tie the ends together. Attach 10 pounds or more of weight to the tied ends of the strip. Lean forward, drape the strip of cloth over the back of your head, and then brace your hands on your knees. Exercise your neck muscles by lifting the weight up and down with your head by extending and flexing your neck. Do twelve to fifteen repetitions.

In addition to strengthening neck muscles, this resistive neck exercise will help restore the normal neck curve when it has been flattened or reversed by years of chronic tension.

Try to do both exercises—shoulder shrugs and neck lifts—every other day, or at least twice a week, for a few months.

How to Relieve the Headache of Hypoglycemia

When you miss a few meals or go without eating for several hours, you might experience a headache caused by hypoglycemia, a drop in blood sugar. This is a normal reaction when it occurs after several hours of not eating. This type of headache is promptly relieved by eating.

There are two other types of hypoglycemia—functional and organic—that are not normal, however. One is caused by pancreatic sensitivity and what you eat and the other is caused by organic disease. It's important that you distinguish between the two so that you'll know when to help yourself and when to see a doctor. Functional hypoglycemia can lead to pancreatic fatigue and diabetes, while organic hypoglycemia may be an indication of a pancreatic tumor.

Functional Hypoglycemia

Eating the wrong kinds of foods commonly results in headache caused by a drop in blood sugar. In functional hypoglycemia, for example, blood sugar falls three to five hours after eating sugar, white flour, and other refined carbohydrates. In susceptible persons, any of the refined carbohydrates, commonly found in processed foods, can be quickly absorbed, overloading the blood with glucose and causing a sensitive or overactive pancreas to produce an excessive amount of insulin. The result is that too much glucose is removed from the blood for storage as glycogen and fat, depriving the brain and the muscles of adequate fuel. This causes headache, fatigue, and a variety of other symptoms.

If you suffer from functional hypoglycemia, you should eat fresh, natural foods in three meals a day and include a low-fat protein snack, such as cottage cheese and fruit or a piece of baked chicken, between meals. If you're not overweight, peanut butter or cheese with whole grain bread or crackers is fine. Sweets and refined carbohydrates should be eliminated or reduced to a minimum. Natural complex carbohydrates, such as fruits, vegetables, and whole grains, are digested and absorbed slowly because of their high fiber content and will not overstimulate your pancreas.

Disease-Caused Organic Hypoglycemia

Persons who suffer from hypoglycemia caused by organic disease, such as a pancreatic tumor, suffer constantly from weakness, shakiness, fatigue, inability to think clearly, and other symptoms of low blood sugar. Symptoms are relieved only temporarily by eating.

Victims of organic hypoglycemia usually wake up in the morning with headache and other hangover-type symptoms that are relieved by breakfast. A victim of functional hypoglycemia, on the other hand, may feel fine before breakfast but will experience symptoms of low blood sugar a few hours after eating such refined carbohydrates as pancakes and syrup.

You can usually relieve or eliminate symptoms of functional hypoglycemia by making a few changes in your eating habits. The persistent symptoms of organic hypoglycemia, however, should always be brought to the attention of a physician.

Your doctor might order a simple fasting blood sugar analysis when he suspects that you are suffering from organic hypoglycemia. Symptoms of functional hypoglycemia call for a glucose tolerance test, in which blood sugar is tested every hour for five hours after drinking a glucose solution.

Remember: In organic hypoglycemia, fasting blood sugar is consistently low, whereas in functional hypoglycemia, the fasting blood sugar may be normal, dropping to a low level a few hours after eating refined carbohydrates or after drinking a sweet beverage.

Be sure to read Chapter 6 for tips on how to eat properly to protect your health and reduce excess body fat so that you can *prevent* the pancreatic sensitivity that leads to functional hypoglycemia. In the process, you'll relieve headache caused by constipation as well as backache caused by being overweight. A good diet with proper nutrition is one of the most important self-help measures you can follow—for a variety of ailments.

How Arnie J. Solved His Problems by Changing His Diet

Arnie J. was a typical victim of functional hypoglycemia. He also suffered from constipation, headache, obesity, and backache. "Every day, in the middle of the morning and in the middle of the afternoon," he reported, "I'm so hungry, weak, and shaky that I can hardly get my work done. And I usually have a headache by the time I get home from work."

All Arnie had to do to feel good again was to make a few simple changes in his diet. Following the dietary guidelines I have outlined in Chapter 6, he had fruit and whole-grain cereal for breakfast instead of his usual pancakes and syrup. For lunch, he switched from coffee and donuts to such fresh, natural foods as fish and vegetables.

"My energy has doubled!" Arnie exclaimed. "I'm feeling great for the first time in years. I've lost 25 pounds, my constipation has been relieved, and I no longer have headaches and backaches. What a wonderful diet!"

The Triangle of Constipation, Headache, and Backache

We all know from experience that constipation can cause headache. Such a headache is not caused by absorption of toxins as once believed, but by a reflex mechanism from pressure in the colon and rectum. Researchers have found, for example, that stuffing the rectum with cotton can trigger a headache in some people.

Failure to empty the bowels regularly leads to rectal stuffing. Delay in evacuation allows absorption of water from waste matter, resulting in impaction of hardened matter in the lower bowel and rectum. This can cause a reflex headache along with all the other discomforts of constipation, including backache.

If you ever suffer an acute, incapacitating attack of back pain, chances are your bowels will temporarily cease functioning, resulting in constipation. Your body simply protects your painful lower back by halting contractions in bowel and abdominal muscles. Generally, the constipation will correct itself when the back pain subsides. But if it persists for more than three or four days, you should make a special effort to aid in the emptying of your lower bowel. A simple enema might be needed to get things started. From there, you can observe the self-help measures outlined in this chapter.

Constipation and Colon Cancer

There is more to be concerned about than headache when you are a victim of chronic constipation. Pouches, or diverticuli, formed by excessive pressures in the colon can eventually become inflamed and spastic, resulting in diverticulitis and hemorrhoids. There is also now considerable evidence to indicate that prolonged retention of waste in the colon can cause colon cancer. The theory is that fecal waste retained too long in the colon allows bacterial activity to convert bile acids to cancer-causing toxins. Today, colon cancer is the second most common cause of death from cancer.

Obviously, even if you are not now suffering from constipation or headache, you should give your bowels the attention they deserve if you want to live a long, comfortable life.

How Frances C. Improved Her Quality of Life by Getting Rid of Her Constipation

Frances C. had suffered from constipation for many years and was literally addicted to laxatives. Straining when on the toilet often caused her hemorrhoids to bleed. Her overloaded colon occasionally inflamed the diverticuli, or small pouches, in her colon, causing painful abdominal cramps that were sometimes accompanied by diarrhea.

"My stomach trouble plays heck with my social life," Frances confided. "I'm often miserable when I go out in the evening. If I don't have a headache, I have cramps in my abdomen."

Frances followed the simple suggestions on the treatment and prevention of constipation. After a few months, she reported that her constipation problem had been solved. "Best of all," she added, "my headaches, hemorrhoids, and abdominal cramps have practically disappeared."

Treating and Preventing Constipation

We all suffer from constipation occasionally. A trip out of town, a change in routine or sleeping hours, stress, and other factors can result in a temporary interruption of bowel habits. Usually, if you eat properly and keep your days and nights regulated, your bowels will take care of themselves, relieving your constipation in a day or two. You should not have to take a laxative or an enema.

Don't jump to the conclusion that you suffer from constipation if you don't have a bowel movement every day, as most people do. While it's usually best to have one or more bowel movements daily, some people do not have daily bowel movements. In fact, it may be perfectly normal for some people to have one only every two days.

If you are accustomed to having a bowel movement every day, and you miss a couple of days, or if your stool becomes hard or is in the shape of marbles, you should make a special effort to empty your bowels. Failure to have a bowel movement over a period of three or four days may allow accumulating waste to become packed and hardened, making evacuation difficult or impossible.

So while you should not panic when your bowels fail to move for a day or two, you should not ignore constipation, and you should make sure that your daily eating and living habits are not contributing to the development of chronic constipation.

Common Causes of Constipation

One of the most common causes of constipation is failure to have a bowel movement on a regular schedule. Busy people often ignore the urge to go, refusing to take the time needed to empty their bowels. The result is that the urge disappears, allowing the bowel to absorb water from the accumulating waste. Then, when the person finally attempts a bowel movement, either the urge is not present or the hardened fecal matter in the rectum blocks the emptying of the colon.

People who take laxatives to force the emptying of their bowels, while failing to take measures to correct the cause of their constipation, often develop the serious problem of *chronic* constipation.

Avoid the Use of Laxatives Whenever Possible

Regular use of laxatives can result in an addiction to laxatives. The bowels simply become accustomed to emptying only when stimulated by a powerful irritant. If you do take a laxative occasionally, remember that when the intestinal tract has been emptied by the artificial stimulation of a laxative, it may take three or four days for enough waste to accumulate in the rectum to trigger an urge to visit the toilet again. So don't become impatient after a day or two and take another laxative, lest your bowels become dependent upon artificial stimulation.

Actually, it would probably be better to take an enema rather than a laxative when the lower bowel is clogged or impacted. An enema will not affect the entire intestinal tract as a laxative does. An enema, like a laxative, will rarely be necessary if you care for your bowels properly, however. If you do become constipated occasionally, your body will handle the problem after a day or two if you eat properly and follow a sensible schedule.

Whatever you do, whether you occasionally take a laxative or an enema or not, there are some basic rules that you should observe every day of your life.

Eliminate Solid Waste on a Regular Schedule

Try to visit the toilet at the same time every day, preferably after eating. Always make sure that you allow enough time for each visit.

Never ignore an urge to empty your bowels, even if the urge occurs at a time you do not normally visit the toilet. Even when your bowels have been emptied in response to an unscheduled urge, you should continue to visit the toilet at your usual times in order to keep yourself regulated.

Eat Fiber-Rich Natural Foods

The type of foods you eat can be very important in the treatment and prevention of constipation. If you eat predominantly refined and processed foods, for example, lack of adequate fiber in your diet will result in dry, concentrated stools that will be difficult to move. Furthermore, the residue of such refined carbohydrates as sugar and white flour products encourages the growth of unfriendly colon bacteria that feed on the slow-moving contents of the bowel, producing cancer-causing toxins.

One of the most important things you must do every day—to protect your health as well as to prevent headache and bowel discomfort—is to eat a variety of fresh, natural fruits, vegetables, and whole-grain products. These natural carbohydrates are rich in the fiber your bowels need for moisture-retaining bulk that will stimulate bowel movements and encourage the growth of *friendly* bacteria. Fiber in your bowels will also sweep intestinal pouches clean, thus preventing diverticulitis.

With the exception of grains, natural carbohydrates are generally high in water. Even a good high-carbohydrate diet, however, should be supplemented with plenty of water each day to make sure that the fiber in your colon retains a maximum amount of moisture. This will assure soft, well-formed stools that can be easily moved.

You should be able to get all the fiber you need from natural carbohydrates. If you are unable to eat properly every day, or if you are having difficulty emptying your bowels, you should add a little miller's bran to your diet. A couple tablespoons of bran added to your morning cereal should be enough. Or, you might prefer to add bran to homemade bread or meat loaf. You can find miller's bran in any health food store. When high-fiber foods are not available, the use of psyllium seed products (with plenty of water) is a beneficial and harmless way to introduce stool-softening bulk into the bowels.

Be sure to read Chapter 6 for additional information on maintainting a high-fiber diet.

HEADACHE BRIEF

Tension headaches are often characterized by tightness in muscles around the head, neck, and shoulders and can often be relieved with massage, stretching, relaxation exercises, moist heat, and over-the-counter pain medication, such as aspirin or acetaminophen (such as Tylenol).

Cluster headaches should be suspected when there is a regularly recurring headache with severe pain behind one eye along with nasal stuffiness and redness in the eyes. This type of headache occurs primarily in men. Trigger factors, such as certain foods, alcohol, and tobacco smoke, should be identified and eliminated. Prescription medication may be needed when pain is frequent and severe.

Sinus headaches typically involve obvious nasal congestion and clogging with pain around one or both eyes. Over-the-counter pain medications with antihistamine-decongestant are often helpful. But when there is fever with green or yellow mucous, there may be an infection, and an antibiotic may be needed.

Migraine headaches are usually preceded by visual disturbances and accompanied by pain on one side of the head along with nausea or vomiting and sensitivity to bright light; migraine may require prescription medication for relief of symptoms. Migraine headaches occur primarily in women.

When You Need Medication

If you have migraine headaches, your doctor might want to prescribe special medication, such as an ergot derivative, to relieve pain caused by dilated and swollen blood vessels around your brain. Special medication might also be prescribed in the treatment and prevention of painful cluster headaches. For most of us, however, simple over-the-counter medication such as acetylsalicylic acid (the ingredient of aspirin, Ecotrin, and Empirin), ibuprofen (such as Advil, Motrin, and Nuprin), acetaminophen (such as Tylenol, Anacin II, and Datril), and other medications containing these ingredients, sometimes in combination with caffeine (as in Excedrin or Vanquish), may be adequate for relief of headache pain.

Over-the-counter drugs can have side effects, however, and should be taken only occasionally. Aspirin, for example, can irritate the stomach and intestines, and it can interfere with blood clotting when taken in large or frequent doses. Prolonged use of aspirin might cause gastrointestinal bleeding. If you are taking a blood thinner or if you have gastritis or a stomach ulcer, you may have to take acetaminophen instead of aspirin.

Acetaminophen will not inflame your stomach or cause bleeding, but excessive or prolonged use of this medication can damage your liver. Remember that discontinuing the use of any headache medication you have been taking for a long time may result in a rebound effect that could make your headache worse.

Be cautious about taking any kind of medication unnecessarily. An occasional aspirin or acetaminophen can provide blessed relief when you are racked with head pain that interferes with sleep. It's always best, however, to first try natural remedies in seeking relief from simple tension headache. Also, it's always a good idea to talk with your family doctor before taking any kind of medication, especially if you have other medical problems.

S U M M A R Y

1. Most headaches are the result of tension and tight neck muscles and can be relieved with simple techniques.

2. Persistent headaches, especially when accompanied by other symptoms, should be brought to the attention of a physician.

3. Moist heat, massage, and a little neck stretching are often an effective combination for relieving headache caused by tight neck muscles.

4. Amines in chocolate, cheese, and wine will sometimes trigger a vascular-type headache in susceptible persons.

5. The sodium nitrite preservative in hot dogs and lunchmeats is a potent vasodilator that can trigger a vascular headache.

6. Monosodium glutamate, salt, and other sodium additives should be avoided if you suspect they are the cause of your headache.

7. If food allergy is a factor in your headaches, you should eliminate the suspected foods from your diet for one month and see if your headache disappears.

8. Stuffy rooms, heater fumes, bright light, stress, noise, and other extreme environmental factors can cause headache and should be controlled or eliminated.

9. Headaches resulting from hypoglycemia caused by eating refined carbohydrates can be eliminated by eating a balanced diet of fresh, natural foods in each of your three daily meals.

10. Headaches caused by constipation can be prevented by eating high-fiber, water-rich natural carbohydrates and by visiting the toilet a couple of times a day on a regular basis.

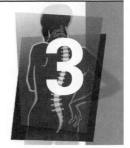

How to Relieve
Neck, Shoulder, and
Arm Pain

Jonathan D., twenty-eight years old, woke one morning with a severe pain on the left side of his neck. The slightest movement caused stabbing pain that seemed to reach from his neck to his shoulder blade. He could turn his head to the right without much difficulty, but attempts to turn his head to the left triggered severe pain and spasm.

"My neck feels as if it is broken," Jonathan complained with a note of panic. "When I move my head, there's a knifelike pain in my neck."

Jonathan spent the day with his head tilted to the right, afraid to move. On the second day, he called my office, convinced that his neck was "out of place." A quick history revealed that Jonathan had no previous history of neck trouble and had never sustained a neck injury. There were also no indications of arthritis or bone disease.

"Let's give it a couple more days before we consider X-raying your neck," I told Jonathan. I instructed him in the use of home treatment methods and told him to call back after three days.

On the third day after visiting my office, Jonathan called. "My neck pain is almost gone," he reported, "and I can turn my head. Those home remedies really did the trick."

Actually, Jonathan's neck problem was not serious—just a simple "crick" or muscle spasm—and would have eventually disappeared no matter what he did. But the home remedies helped. And such remedies can very often mean the difference between a speedy recovery and a long, miserable siege.

The Different Sources of Neck Pain

There are seven vertebrae in the neck, forming a canal that houses the brain stem and the spinal cord. Blood vessels pass up through the neck and the cervical spine, forming a network of blood vessels at the base of the brain, supplying brain tissues with blood flow and oxygen. Nerve centers in the brain stem near the top of the cervical spine supply important respiratory muscles. Nerves passing down from the brain stem through the spinal cord supply all the musculoskeletal structures in the body from the neck down.

With the cervical vertebrae joined together in a fashion that permits the head and neck to move in almost every imaginable direction, the cervical spine is an extremely delicate and important structure. Although lower back trouble may be the most common cause of disability, neck injury is potentially more serious. Obviously, it's just as important to pay as much attention to your neck as to your lower back. Fortunately, everyday neck problems are rarely serious.

Muscle spasms or minor joint injuries, such as the neck crick Jonathan experienced, are often caused by bad sleeping posture or an awkward movement. They can trigger neck pain that is not nearly as serious as it feels. Usually, the pain and spasm will subside after four or five days, and it won't be necessary to undergo a potentially harmful X-ray examination or drug treatment.

There are, of course, many causes of neck pain, and some could be serious. Any neck pain that persists, is accompanied by other symptoms, has been preceded by injury, or is associated with disease should be brought to the attention of a physician. See Chapter 1 for ways to pinpoint the cause of your pain.

In this chapter, we'll discuss some of the common causes of neck, shoulder, and arm pain and what you can do about them at home.

How to Handle the Common Neck Crick

A neck crick, a painful muscle spasm or locking of the neck, is a common neck problem. Doctors do not know what causes cricks. Fatigue, postural strain, and drafts of cold air can sometimes trigger the muscle spasm of a crick. Pulled muscles, joint injuries, misalignment of vertebrae, pinching of joint capsules, and disc protrusions are also often blamed for an acutely locked neck.

Occasionally, a joint in the neck will bind or lock to cause a painful locking of the neck. When this occurs, a single manipulation by a chiropractor, an osteopath, or a physiatrist will often unlock the involved joint, resulting in immediate relief. Most of the time, however, it is muscle spasm that locks the neck, and this is usually the result of an injury to a muscle attachment, a joint surface, or a joint capsule. Such spasm simply will not go away until the injury subsides or heals, which takes a little time. So don't panic the next time you wake up with a neck crick. Chances are it will subside or disappear in a few days if you combine time with a few home remedies.

Sleeping soundly in an awkward position seems to be the most common cause of injuries that result in neck cricks. If you happen to have arthritis or some other problem in the joints of your neck, you may be even more susceptible to recurrences of muscle spasms in your neck. Deep sleep, such as that induced by alcohol or extreme fatigue, overcomes protective reflexes and allows joints to sag unprotected in bad sleeping postures, straining sensitive muscles, joints, and ligaments.

Because the pain of a neck spasm can be severe and because unrelieved muscle spasm can prolong symptoms and delay recovery, there are a few basic treatments that you should try at home.

Rest Is Important

When a neck muscle is in spasm, try to get as much rest as you can to relieve tension on already tight neck muscles. Lie down occasionally or shorten your working day so that your neck muscles are not overly fatigued. Neck muscles that are in spasm fatigue easily. If they are forced to hold your head in a fatiguing posture for very long, the added tension will increase the spasm. This will result in an accumulation of lactic acid waste products that will inflame muscles and produce more spasm.

A Cervical Collar Might Help

When a neck spasm is overworked by postural strain, the neck muscles become so fatigued that they might not be able to hold your head up. When this happens and it's not possible to rest, a simple soft cervical collar, available in any drugstore, might help you get through the day. The collar will provide a surface to rest your chin on so that you can continue to look straight ahead without depending totally upon fatigued neck muscles.

How Bennett J. Relieved His Neck Pain by Using
a Cervical Collar

Bennett J., a state legislator, walked into my office one day complaining of neck spasm that had persisted throughout a week of legislative meetings. His neck muscles had become so fatigued that he could barely keep his chin off his chest. "I have another week of meetings scheduled," Bennett explained. "I need a little help to get through the week."

I recommended a soft cervical collar for Bennett and told him to wear it only as a temporary aid during the day—until the legislature adjourned. When he returned for physical therapy a week later, his neck was much improved. "The collar helped greatly," he reported. "It rested my neck enough that I began to improve immediately." After a few days of therapy, he was doing fine.

Most of the time, you can avoid wearing a cervical collar for a stiff neck if you get adequate rest and use such simple home remedies as moist heat.

Moist Heat Relaxes Muscles

Moist heat is usually the most effective treatment for muscle spasms and cricks. As you learned in Chapter 2, you can apply moist heat to your neck by standing under a hot shower, by applying hot, wet towels to your neck, or by wrapping your neck with a roll of flannel-covered hot, wet towels.

You should *never* sleep with a heating pad; you could suffer a burn. You should always limit heat applications to fifteen or twenty minutes, repeated every two or three hours as needed.

Moist heat applications can be kept hot with a hot-water bottle, an insulated heating pad (use these carefully and follow the directions provided by the manufacturer), or the rays of an infrared bulb. You can purchase a moist-heat heating pad that you simply moisten under a faucet before turning on the heat.

How to Use Cold to Relieve Pain

Some doctors recommend cold applications (cryotherapy) for painful neck and back problems. Since cold relieves pain but does not speed healing, I usually recommend a trial with moist heat in the treatment of neck spasms and cricks. If heat does not relieve the pain by relaxing the muscles, cold may then be tried for pain relief.

You can apply cold to the neck by using damp towels that have been chilled in a refrigerator, by rubbing the affected muscles with a cylinder of ice, or by applying an ice-filled Ziploc bag that has been covered with a moist hand towel. Or you may simply use a commercial ice bag or refrigerated cold pack.

When ice is applied to a painful area, it may take from five to fifteen minutes to numb the pain. When the skin is numb and the pain has subsided, the ice should be removed within three minutes. Remember that excessive or prolonged application of cold can damage tissues.

How to Use Ice Massage

The best way to make a cylinder of ice for ice massage is to freeze water in a paper cup and then peel away the paper. An ice cream stick can be frozen into the water to serve as a handle. Running a little hot water over the cup of frozen water will facilitate removal of the paper.

The painful area of the neck should be rubbed with ice for several minutes, until the pain has been numbed by cold. Before numbness occurs, there will be a feeling of warmth followed by a burning sensation. The ice massage should be discontinued when the skin feels numb. Once the pain is relieved, it might be possible to unlock your neck by turning your head from side to side.

Heat Versus Cold for Pain Relief

Generally, cold is more effective than heat in relieving throbbing pain caused by acute inflammation and swelling. In such injuries as a pulled muscle, a bruise, or a sprain, you should always use cold. When obvious bleeding and swelling are present, as in torn muscles or ligaments, cold should be used for three or four days before trying heat. In the case of a neck crick, however, there is usually little or no swelling and very little inflammation during the first day or two. For this reason, it's always best to try muscle-relaxing heat before trying cold when you wake up with a spasm in your neck.

When you do use cold to relieve the pain and spasm of a neck crick, you should switch to moist heat a day or two after the pain has subsided in order to warm and relax muscles and flush them with a fresh flow of blood. Prolonged or excessive use of cold might actually inflame muscles by depriving them of adequate blood flow. When blood flow is restricted by a fifteen- or twenty-minute application of cold, circulation *increases* a few hours later if the cold application is not repeated. This is why cold applications are applied every two to four hours for twenty-four to seventy-two hours when there is severe swelling. Remember, however, that excessive use of cold can result in the *spasm* of blood vessels, depriving tissues of adequate oxygen. So don't use cold continuously or for longer than three or four days.

Cold *restricts* circulation (during application) to relieve pain caused by swelling and inflammation. Heat speeds healing by *increasing* circulation. When in doubt about which to use, always use cold the first day or two, especially if there has been an injury. When there has not been an injury, as in the case of an early morning neck crick, you may simply experiment with cold and heat and then use whichever feels best to you. When heat does not seem to help, or if it increases pain, try cold. Even when there is no swelling, cold can relieve pain by numbing nerves.

How a Pillow Can Either Support or Strain Your Neck

Since most neck cricks seem to develop during sleep, the position of your head while sleeping may have much to do with the development of neck spasm. Sleeping with your head on a pillow that is too high, too low, or too soft, for example, may place damaging strain on the muscles and joints of your neck. A high pillow may lift your head too high, stretching and reversing the normal curve of your neck. A pillow that is too thin for persons who have a back hump may allow the head to tilt backward, jamming joints and pinching nerves. A small pillow that supports your head and not your neck may allow your neck vertebrae to sag, straining joints and ligaments.

A pillow that is too soft and spongy may cause some sleepers to push back against the springy support of the pillow, forcing unconscious contraction of neck muscles.

Even when you have a good pillow, lying with your head rolled to one side and half off the pillow may place a strain on joints and muscle attachments in your neck, especially if you are sleeping too soundly to wake up in response to discomfort. It's important to have a good sleeping posture as well as a good pillow. Chapter 9 provides more information about sleeping postures.

Which Pillows Are Best?

There are many neck or "cervical pillows" on the market; some are good and some are bad. Cervical rolls that support only the neck can be bad, since they may place too much pressure directly against the joints of the neck. Solid, molded pillows fit some persons and not others. A molded

Figure 3-1. Fluffing up the bottom edge of a thin pillow so that the back of the neck and the back of the head are equally supported will help maintain normal alignment of the cervical spine.

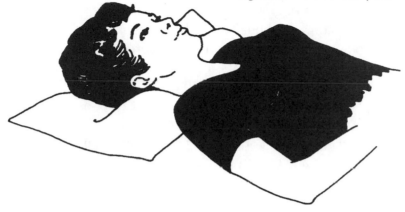

pillow that's good for sleeping on your back may not be suitable for sleeping on your side. If you are a wide-shouldered person, for example, you may need a thin pillow while sleeping on your back and a thick pillow while sleeping on your side.

Persons with a humped or slumped spine may have to have an extra-thick pillow to keep their head from tilting backward when sleeping on their back. Obviously, no one pillow will fit everyone's needs. *Whatever type of pillow you use, it should support both your head and your neck so that your neck is relaxed and aligned with the rest of your spine.* There should be no tilting, sagging, bending, or rotation in your neck vertebrae.

Regardless of the position you assume, the pillow you use should support your head and your neck equally. If you're shaped like the average person, the part of the pillow supporting your neck should be a little thicker than the part of the pillow supporting your head.

I usually advise my patients to buy old-fashioned pillows that are thick or thin enough to meet their individual needs. The part of the pillow supporting your neck can be fluffed up to fit into the contour of the neck.

In addition to causing neck pain, an inappropriate pillow can cause headache by interfering with sleep and placing tension on your neck. So even if you don't suffer from neck cricks, there are other reasons you should protect your neck by selecting a pillow that is appropriate for you and your sleeping posture. With the right pillow, you can prevent some types of headache and neck pain and avoid aggravating old neck problems.

Slipped Discs and Pinched Nerves

When neck pain persists or grows worse after several days, or when pain radiates down your arm, you should see a physician for a diagnosis of your problem. The older you become, the more important it will be to seek a specific diagnosis, since age brings a greater variety of both Type M (mechanical) and Type O (organic) disorders that can cause neck and arm pain. Older persons, for example, are more subject to bone and arterial diseases that might require specific medical care.

Most of the time, persistent or recurring neck pain is caused by deterioration of disc cartilage and by arthritic changes, which can result in irritation of a spinal nerve.

Normally, there is ample room for the spinal nerves that pass between the vertebrae. When a disc ruptures or degenerates, however, or when arthritic spurs form, these abnormal changes result in the pinching of sensitive spinal nerves. This may cause pain that radiates into the shoulder, down the arm, or into two or three fingers. Such pain is often accompanied by numbness, tingling, and other symptoms, which doctors call radiculitis.

The pain of a pinched nerve is generally severe and can result in sensory disturbance or muscle weakness in the portion of the arm supplied by the affected nerve, causing radiculopathy, or nerve damage. Evidence of progressive nerve damage includes muscle shrinkage or a diminished tendon reflex, and it is important that you see a neurologist if these symptoms occur. Regularly compare one arm with the other. If portions of the painful arm appear to be getting smaller, that may be a sign of nerve damage.

How to Handle a Pinched Nerve

Most of the time, you will recover from a pinched nerve. Your body may build up scar tissue to protect nerves irritated by spurs. Herniated discs will degenerate with time, removing the painful protrusion that's too close to a spinal nerve. Sometimes, the pain of a pinched nerve will be relieved when the swelling in the involved disc and nerve subsides. If there is no progressive nerve damage taking place, you may be able to use rest and home remedies to relieve symptoms, thus buying the time your body needs to heal itself.

When arm pain is persistent or unrelieved, you should be examined periodically by a physician who can check deep tendon reflexes, sensory ability, and muscle strength in the part of the arm supplied by the affected nerve. If there is evidence to indicate that nerve damage may weaken the affected shoulder, arm, or hand, a neurosurgeon or an orthopedist might recommend removal of the offending spur or disc protrusion. Always seek a second opinion if this is advised. Ask why surgery is being recommended and if it is necessary. Weigh the consequences of refusing surgery as opposed to submitting to surgery. Spinal disc surgery is sometimes clearly indicated and sometimes it is not. If there is no progressive nerve damage and no MRI evidence of a massive disc protrusion compressing a spinal nerve, ask about alternatives. You might be able to use moist heat, cold packs, rest, neck traction, appropriate pillows, and simple medications to relieve pain and aid recovery. A soft cervical collar might help guard against nerve root irritation.

TABLE OF PINCHED NECK NERVES

A pinched nerve in the neck will refer pain, numbness, and other symptoms into certain portions of the head, neck, shoulder, or arm. Listed here are the cervical vertebra and the areas that each supplies:

- **C1** (the uppermost vertebra in the neck) supplies the top of the head.

- **C2** supplies the skin and muscles on the front and back of the head.

- **C3** supplies each side of the head and neck.

- **C4** supplies structures across the shoulder and upper back area.

- **C5** supplies portions of the shoulder and upper arm.

- **C6** reaches down the arm into thumb and index finger.

- **C7** passes down the arm into long and ring fingers.

- **C8** reaches into the little finger (along with the ring finger, occasionally).

Note: Although the spinal nerves from C5 through C8 supply certain structures as they pass down the arm, the nerve affected is best identified by symptoms at the end point of the nerve.

The Potential Benefits and Drawbacks of Manipulation

Manipulation of vertebrae, when performed by a chiropractor or an osteopath, will sometimes relieve neck pain and symptoms of nerve root irritation. Such treatment might aggravate symptoms caused by compression of a spinal nerve, however. If cervical manipulation does not seem to help after a few treatments, or if it seems to make the pain worse, manipulation should stop.

Cervical manipulation is potentially dangerous. In rare instances, forceful rotation of the cervical spine combined with extension might damage vertebral arteries or rupture weakened blood vessels at the base of the brain, causing a stroke. Although the American Chiropractic Association (Arlington, VA) maintains that the benefits of properly performed cervical manipulation outweigh any possible risks, the National Council Against Health Fraud (www.ncahf.org) warns that there is not sufficient evidence to justify the risk of cervical manipulation under any circumstances.

If you find that occasional cervical manipulation seems to relieve your neck pain or your tension headache, you should undergo such treatment only after careful preliminary screening and with informed consent.

Although manipulation, or adjustment of the vertebrae, is often touted as a method of relieving pinched nerves, a nerve that is truly pinched by a spur or a disc herniation is very unlikely to respond well to manipulation. In fact, in some cases, the presence of nerve root impingement is a good reason to avoid the use of manipulation, especially if one treatment results in a painful reaction.

When a joint is stiffened by fixations or locked by spasm and misalignment, one or two manipulations may provide dramatic relief. But forced movement of a diseased joint that is pinching a nerve may do more harm than good. Of course, a competent chiropractor or osteopath will use cervical manipulation cautiously and only in appropriate cases.

Avoid Unnecessary Manipulation

When manipulation does relieve neck pain or arm pain, the manipulation should be discontinued when the pain is gone. Continued use of cervical manipulation as a preventive measure might actually result in a recurrence of symptoms, not to mention the risk of injury to vascular structures in your neck. I tell my patients, "If your neck doesn't hurt, leave it alone."

Don't become a permanent patient by submitting to regular spinal manipulation to prevent symptoms you don't have. Unnecessary and excessive use of manipulation could result in the need for manipulation to relieve symptoms *caused* by the manipulation.

Some chiropractic patients are convinced that regular spinal "adjustments" will prevent the development of organic disease by keeping the vertebrae in proper alignment. This is a theory and is not supported by scientific consensus. An occasional manipulation to loosen vertebrae between your shoulders and in your lower back will probably make you feel better, but I doubt that such treatment will improve your health or prolong your life, as claimed by some chiropractors. I have patients who come for spinal manipulation because it feels good and because it relieves tension, but only occasionally and not for organic problems.

How to Relieve Neck and Arm Pain by Stretching Your Neck at Home

Use of cervical traction—or neck stretching—at home will often provide relief from neck and arm pain caused by disc degeneration and arthritis. If your doctor recommends neck traction, you can purchase a cervical traction apparatus in any surgical supply store or in a drugstore that sells home health supplies. Some drugstores will supply cervical traction equipment without a prescription.

Sitting cervical traction is the type of traction most often prescribed for use at home. In some cases, however, neck traction is more effective when lying down—the way it is done in most hospitals. You may have to determine for yourself which orientation works the best for you. If you are using sitting cervical traction and your arm pain is not improving or is getting worse, try switching to traction while lying down. In my office, I usually try both types of traction on the patient before prescribing home traction.

In either type of traction, sitting or lying down, there should be some immediate relief from pain. If the traction is uncomfortable, or if it increases the pain, then you're either using too much weight, using the wrong type of traction, using it improperly, or staying in it too long. Or maybe you should not be using it at all. Discontinue use of traction if it makes your pain worse.

3

How to Rig Up Sitting Cervical Traction

A sitting cervical traction apparatus usually consists of overhead pulleys and a harness that fits around your head and under your chin. A weight is attached to a cord that runs from the harness and over the pulleys. Usually, the pulleys are fastened to a bracket that can be hooked over the top of an open door. You simply sit in a chair or on a stool with your back to the door so that the weight hangs suspended behind you while you are wearing the head harness.

When traction is appropriate and used properly, the steady pull on your neck will stretch tight neck muscles and relieve nerve pressure by pulling the vertebrae of your neck slightly apart.

Selecting the Correct Amount of Weight

When you first begin to use neck traction, try using around seven pounds for ten or fifteen minutes. If no ill effects occur, try using 10 or 12 pounds for fifteen minutes or longer. If you do not experience any relief from pain, you may try using a heavier weight for a shorter period of time or a lighter weight for a longer period of time. For example, you may use 15 or more pounds for ten minutes or less, or you may use 7 or more pounds for an hour or longer.

Be guided by the way you feel. Select the amount of weight that feels best for you and then use it as often or as long as necessary to provide relief from pain. Some patients report relief with as much as 20 pounds for several seconds at a time.

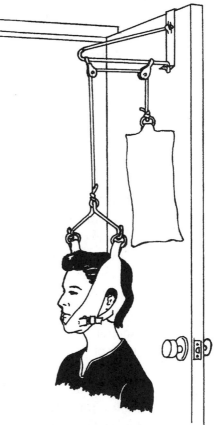

Figure 3-2. *Simple neck stretching at home, using a cervical traction harness, will sometimes relieve neck, shoulder, and arm pain.*

64 ■ THE CHIROPRACTOR'S SELF-HELP BACK AND BODY BOOK

Whenever you begin to experience discomfort during traction, either reduce the amount of weight you're using or decrease the time. If the weight is too heavy or the time too long, your neck muscles will tense up in resistance to the traction. It's important that your neck muscles be as relaxed as possible so that your spine will be stretched. This can sometimes be accomplished better with a lighter weight than with a heavier weight.

How Roger T. Used Neck Traction to Relieve His Pain

Roger T. came into my office complaining of neck, shoulder, and arm pain that was accompanied by numbness and tingling in his forearm, thumb, and forefinger. An X-ray examination revealed that a degenerating disc between the fifth and the sixth cervical vertebrae was allowing the two arthritic vertebrae to come too close together, irritating the sixth cervical spinal nerve. I recommended cervical traction for Roger and suggested that he use it at home.

Roger experienced complete relief from pain while the traction was being applied. It took several weeks of regular use of traction before the pain and numbness were completely gone.

"I used the traction twice a day, about fifteen or twenty minutes each time," Roger reported. "Most of the time, I used about 12 pounds. My arm has quit hurting and I feel as good as new."

Sitting cervical traction is convenient for people who want to use traction in their office or while traveling. The door pulley and the head harness can be easily transported and used anywhere there is a door. A plastic bag filled with water makes a good travel weight. Cervical traction is safe when it is comfortable. It should not be used when it causes discomfort of any kind.

Traction while Lying in Bed

For some persons, traction while lying down is the best way to relieve arm pain originating in the neck. In some cases, for example, cervical traction must pull with the cervical spine slightly flexed (tilting your chin toward your chest). The only way you can do this while your neck muscles are relaxed is to lie on your back with your head supported by a thick pillow so that the traction pulls uphill about 15 degrees. Special cervical traction apparatus devices that can be attached to a mattress or to a footboard are available at medical/surgical supply stores. Ask for information on how to use the apparatus when you purchase it. A prescription might be required for purchase of a bed traction apparatus.

Home Care for Shoulder Bursitis, Arthritis, and Tendonitis

Neal R. called my office for an appointment. "I think I have a pinched nerve," he said. "I can hardly lift my arm, and the pain is getting worse."

When Neal came into my office, it quickly became apparent that his shoulder and upper arm pain was coming from his shoulder and not from his neck. I examined his neck and his tendon reflexes to make sure that his neck was not involved. Overhead movement of his arm was restricted by shoulder pain rather than by weakness. Significantly, he could not reach behind his back with the affected arm. The diagnosis was supraspinatus tendonitis.

Generally, with tendonitis, or inflammation of a shoulder tendon, movement of the arm will be restricted only in the direction involving use of the affected tendon. Impingement syndrome occurs when swelling of an inflamed tendon that wedges under bony processes in the shoulder prevents elevation of the arm out to the side.

The pain of bursitis, an inflammation of the lubricating sac surrounding the shoulder socket, will restrict movement in all directions, often with extreme pain on the slightest movement.

Arthritis, which is an inflammation of bony surfaces, may result in painful (but not severely painful) movement in all directions without restriction in range of motion. Most victims of shoulder arthritis, for example, can usually lift their arm overhead with slow, painful movement.

Whatever the cause of your shoulder pain, there are some basic self-help measures you can use to relieve pain and improve range of motion while preventing the development of adhesions in the tendons, bursa, or joint. Adhesions are like scar tissue; once they occur, they may have to be stretched with exercise or torn loose by manipulation.

Arm Slings and Cold Packs for Acute Shoulder Pain

When shoulder pain is so acute that the slightest movement causes excruciating pain, it might be necessary to wear an arm sling for a few days. Any drugstore can supply you with an arm sling that can be adjusted to support your arm at a level where there will be no tug on painful shoulder tendons.

It might also be necessary to use heat or a cold pack to relieve the pain. When bursitis is acute, the use of heat may increase the pain. Simple trial and error will quickly tell you which is most effective for pain relief—heat or cold.

If you don't have an ice bag, you can fill a Ziploc bag with crushed ice. You can also make a flexible form-fitting ice pack by mixing three cups of water with one cup of rubbing alcohol in a plastic bag and freezing the mixture to a slush. Or you could simply use a bag of frozen peas. Both can be refrozen for use again and again.

A bag of slush or crushed ice or a bag of frozen peas can be wrapped in a dry towel and applied to the shoulder for about twenty minutes every hour until the pain is relieved. In severe cases, it might be necessary for your physician to inject your shoulder with pain-relieving anti-inflammatory medication.

After acute shoulder pain has subsided, heat might feel better than cold. Apply moist heat for about fifteen minutes three or four times a day. A simple way to do this is to drape a hot, wet towel over your shoulder, then keep it hot with an infrared heat lamp or bulb.

Preserving Range of Motion with Exercise

You can prevent adhesions in a painful shoulder by moving the shoulder through the various ranges of motion as far as pain permits. To begin with, you may not be able to do more than swing your arm. As freedom from pain permits, however, begin moving your arm through a full range of movement in every direction.

- **The pendulum exercise:** Bend forward at your waist and brace your good arm on a chair seat. Let your bad arm hang relaxed. Move your body a little to start your arm swinging like a pendulum, first back and forth and then from side to side. Swing your arm several times in each direction. Keep your muscles relaxed so that your arm hangs like dead weight, with arm movement resulting solely from the momentum generated by body movement. Do this exercise a couple of times a day in order to keep tendons and bursae loose and lubricated.

- **The arm-lift exercise:** As soon as you are able, lift the affected arm overhead as high as you can. Use the opposite arm to push the painful arm up a little higher. Stop when you feel pain. Do this exercise several times a day, striving to lift your arm a little higher each day.

- **The wall exercise:** Stand with your back against a wall and your arms next to your body. Bend your elbows until your forearms are at a right angle to your body and parallel to the floor. Keeping your elbows next to your body and against the wall, rotate your upper arms by moving your forearms from in front of your body sideways to the wall next to your body. Try to touch the wall with your knuckles.

- **The shoulder-extender exercise:** Stand or sit with your hands clasped behind your head. Move your elbows as far back as possible, squeezing your shoulder blades together.

Restoring Range of Motion with a Pulley

In the early stages of tendonitis, before adhesions develop, movement involving active use of the muscles may be more painful than passive movement in which one arm is lifted by the other arm or a device, without using the affected arm's muscles. When this is the case, a pulley can be used to lift the arm overhead without the pain of muscle contraction pulling on inflamed tendons, thus allowing you to do range of motion movements until the pain subsides.

If adhesions do develop, it may be necessary to use an overhead pulley to *forcefully* restore a full range of movement—slowly, over a long period of time.

How Caroline T. Regained the Use of Her Arm by Using a Shoulder Pulley

Caroline T. had suffered from shoulder pain for several weeks. Although the pain had subsided somewhat, she could not lift her arm high enough to comb her hair. "I cannot even reach back to zip my dress," she complained. "If a door or something jerks my arm, the pain just about kills me!"

I told Caroline how to use moist heat and how to perform the range-of-motion exercises described in this chapter. I also drew a diagram showing how to rig a shoulder pulley. She had to work with the exercises and the pulley for several weeks before she was able to regain full use of her shoulder.

"I was beginning to think that my shoulder was going to be permanently stiff," she confessed, "but by using the pulley I was finally able to pull my arm all the way up."

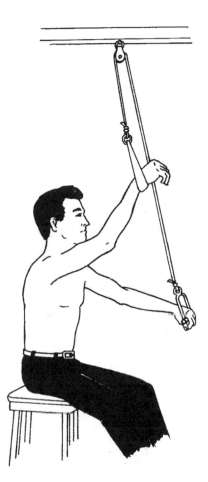

Figure 3-3. *This shoulder pulley exercise can be used to restore or improve range of motion in a stiff or painful shoulder.*

If you have bursitis or tendonitis, you should do all you can to *prevent* the development of adhesions that might freeze your shoulder socket. Do range-of-motion exercises every day. Rig up a pulley the minute you discover that you cannot lift your arm all the way over your head.

How to Rig a Shoulder Pulley

Attach a pulley to the top of a doorway. Run a long piece of sash cord or plastic clothesline over the pulley. Place a chair under the pulley and sit down. Loop one end of the line around the wrist of your bad arm and then reach up and grip the loose end of the line with your good arm. Pull down on the line with your good arm so that the bad arm is hoisted over your head as far as pain will permit.

Use the pulley several times a day until you're able to lift your arm all the way overhead without the assistance of the pulley.

When Elbow Pain Occurs

Elbow pain, like shoulder pain, can originate in the neck. So when you have elbow pain, make sure that it's your elbow and not your neck that needs treatment. When elbow pain is originating in the joints or tendons of the elbow, it should be readily apparent that the elbow is at fault. Bending the elbow or gripping with the hand, for example, may increase pain in the elbow. When elbow pain is referred from the cervical spine, movement or use of the elbow or the hand will not affect the pain.

How Malcolm B. Used Home Remedies to Ease His Elbow Pain

Malcolm B. complained of elbow pain that was greatly aggravated when he tried to turn a doorknob, shake hands, or grip a pair of pliers. He could not even pick up a cup of coffee without elbow pain. "The pain started when I used a screw driver to assemble a book case," he explained.

Malcolm had epicondylitis, or tennis elbow, which is an inflammation of tendon attachments in the elbow. Tendonitis can be caused by any activity that calls for vigorous use of the forearm, as in playing tennis, wringing out clothes, hammering nails, squeezing pliers, and so on. Usually, the problem can be relieved by avoiding painful movements and using moist heat. Malcolm treated his elbow by alternating hot and cold applications. He also wrapped his forearm with a "tennis elbow strap" (just below the painful knob of his elbow). You can find such a strap in most drugstores.

"I was much improved after wearing the strap for three weeks," Malcolm reported, attributing his recovery primarily to use of the strap.

Diagnosing and Treating Persistent Elbow Pain

Once tendonitis develops, it's difficult to cure and may last for months. The pain of tendonitis will usually eventually subside, however. Once you are confident that the correct diagnosis has been made, the time required for recovery shouldn't alarm you.

There are, of course, a variety of conditions that can affect the elbow, some of which must be treated medically. Arthritis, bursitis, gout, and similar conditions, for example, commonly cause pain and swelling in the elbow. All of these conditions, like tendonitis, can cause pain on movement and are sensitive to touch. Your doctor might have to order an X-ray examination and a blood test to differentiate tendonitis from other diseases of the elbow.

With any type of acute elbow pain, an ice pack might be helpful in relieving pain, especially when the pain follows strain or injury. Some athletes treat a painful elbow by slipping a section of inner tube over the elbow and then immersing the rubber-covered joint in a pan of ice water.

As with other joints, moist heat may be more effective in speeding recovery after the acute, initial pain has subsided. Try submerging your elbow in a basin of hot water for about five minutes. While doing this, maintain the temperature by adjusting the water flow to the desired temperature and letting the faucet run just fast enough so that it doesn't exceed the rate of overflow.

When you have elbow pain that is increased by gripping objects, try wrapping your forearm just below the knobs of your elbow. An elastic strap secured around the upper part of your forearm will anchor muscle attachments so there will be less painful pulling at your elbow joint.

If your doctor makes a diagnosis of gout, you may need special medication to keep the disease under control if diet fails to prevent a recurrence of symptoms. You'll learn more about gout in Chapter 8.

Special Wrist and Hand Problems

You already know that persistent pain, numbness, and tingling in a few fingers of one hand often originates in the neck. Whenever this is the case, stretching your neck at home might relieve the symptoms.

Temporary numbness on the little-finger side of your hand and forearm can result from prolonged sitting and lying postures in which there is pressure against the ulnar nerve on the inside of the elbow. Sitting with your arm draped over the back of a chair can compress nerves on the inside of your upper arm, causing weakness in extending your wrist.

Usually, symptoms caused by temporary pressure on nerves in the elbow or upper arm will disappear with time. Be careful, however, not to get yourself into the position of a person I know who developed "Saturday night paralysis." He suffered damage to the nerve supplying his wrist and hand when he fell asleep drunk while his arm was draped over the back of a park bench.

Carpal Tunnel Syndrome

Occasionally, a nerve will be pinched or irritated in the wrist and will cause wrist pain along with numbness, tingling, and weakness in the thumb and first two fingers. This condition is becoming increasingly common because of repetitive trauma to the wrists of persons who operate the keyboards of computers all day. In advanced cases, weakness can be so pronounced that it may not even be possible to grasp a pen or pencil strongly enough to write. When this happens, your doctor might recommend surgery to relieve pressure on the nerve in order to prevent further damage.

Vitamin B-6 (pyridoxine) is sometimes used as a treatment for carpal tunnel syndrome. There is evidence to indicate that B-6 raises the level of a blood enzyme that helps reduce inflammation and swelling in tendons and synovial membranes. Doses should not be higher than one hundred milligrams a day. Researchers have cautioned that two hundred milligrams or more of vitamin B-6 have been associated with some cases of nerve damage; doses of two thousand milligrams or more have caused irreversible nerve damage.

If you have pain, numbness, and tingling in your hands and fingers, keep in touch with your physician to make sure that progressive nerve damage is not taking place. A neurologist can locate and monitor nerve damage by using a special testing procedure called electromyography (EMG).

How Patricia R. Avoided Surgery for Carpal Tunnel Syndrome

Patricia R. had been experiencing pain and numbness in her wrists and hands for several months. She also had numbness and tingling in the thumb, index, and long fingers of both hands. Her symptoms were usually worse at night.

"I thought I had arthritis and that I could live with it," she recalled, "until I began to notice that my hands were getting weak. Now my fingers are so weak that I'm having trouble threading a needle. Sometimes I drop and break wet plates when I'm washing dishes. I'm really afraid that I'm losing the use of my hands."

Patricia was so weak in her thumb and forefinger that she could hardly pick up a book. I had her examined by a neurologist, who confirmed my diagnosis of carpal tunnel syndrome. Electromyography detected pinching of the median nerve between the carpal bones of her wrist where inflammation was present. Instead of immediately submitting to surgery, she used moist heat and cold packs at home, took a 50-milligram vitamin B-6 supplement for a few months, and wore a wrist splint at night. "The treatment is working," she reported on her second visit to my office. "The numbness and tingling are almost gone, and my hands are getting stronger. I'm able to sew a bit now, and I haven't broken a dish in two weeks."

Wrist splints are usually worn at night to relieve pain and reduce pressure on the median nerve by keeping the wrist in a neutral position. The splint may be worn during the day when activities permit and it seems to relieve pain.

In many cases, the symptoms of carpal tunnel syndrome will subside with rest and avoidance of the activity that triggered the symptoms. When there is wrist pain associated with swelling and pain on movement of the wrist, your doctor may have to rule out rheumatoid or gouty arthritis.

Warning: If you develop discoloration in your fingers along with numbness, tingling, or a burning sensation, do not apply cold or extreme heat to your hand or wrist. See your doctor immediately. You might be experiencing the vascular spasm of Raynaud's disease, especially if you are a smoker. The cause of Raynaud's disease, which occurs most often in young women, is unknown. The vascular spasm that deprives the tips of fingers and toes of adequate blood flow can be aggravated by the vasoconstricting effects of nicotine.

SUMMARY

1. Most neck "cricks" will disappear after four or five days, but when symptoms radiate down your arm, you should see a doctor.

2. Ice massage, moist heat, and neck stretching at home will often relieve the pain, spasm, and referred symptoms of an acutely locked neck.

3. Pillows used while sleeping should support your head and neck evenly and keep your neck in line with the rest of your spine, whatever position you're in.

4. Pain radiating from your neck into your arm usually means that a spur or a disc protrusion is pinching or irritating a nerve, requiring rest and cervical traction for recovery.

5. Manipulation will often relieve neck problems, but you should not submit to repeated neck manipulation when symptoms are no longer present, if the treatment does not seem to help, or if it causes pain or discomfort.

6. When you use neck traction at home, try it lying down and sitting up to determine which is most effective for you.

7. Shoulder and upper arm pain that is aggravated by movement of the shoulder joint could be tendonitis, arthritis, or bursitis, all of which can be treated at home with cold packs, moist heat, and range-of-motion exercises.

8. Referred pain in the elbow should not be confused with arthritis, tendonitis, or other conditions that require treatment of the elbow rather than the neck.

9. Sitting or sleeping with pressure on the inside of your elbow or against the inside of your upper arm can result in numbness, tingling, and weakness in your hand and wrist.

10. Carpal tunnel syndrome, in which a pinched nerve in the wrist causes pain, tingling, and weakness in the thumb and first two fingers, can sometimes be relieved by taking vitamin B-6 and wearing a wrist splint.

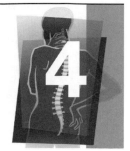

What You Can Do about Back, Hip, and Leg Pain

There are five lumbar vertebrae in the lower spine, with the bottom vertebra sitting on an immobile sacral base, forming the lumbosacral joint. Because of the pressure placed on the lower back and the lumbosacral area, strain most often occurs at this level. With the pounds per square inch pressure much greater in the lower spine than above, disc herniations occur more often there, and lower back trouble is usually more incapacitating than other types of back or neck trouble.

Mechanical abnormalities are common in the lower spine and often complicate a lumbosacral strain. The discs, or cushions, between the vertebrae at the bottom of the spine are larger, thicker, and more likely to rupture or bulge, encroaching upon spinal nerves that supply musculoskeletal structures in the hips, thighs, legs, and feet. Because of the heavy load endured by the lower back, injury, mechanical abnormalities, and ruptured discs often result in structural instability and degenerative changes, triggering the development of arthritis.

Obviously, a little back trouble can lead to more back trouble, making a complete recovery unlikely, often leading to *chronic* back trouble. But there is plenty you can do to protect your back from strain. When you do injure your back, most of what must be done to relieve your pain and speed your recovery can be done at home. And when back trouble is chronic, use of self-help measures such as those outlined in this book will be essential.

4

Time Is on Your Side!

Time is the biggest healer of simple, acute, nonspecific back pain. About 70 percent of all back injuries will resolve in two weeks without any form of treatment; 90 percent will resolve in about four weeks. If you develop leg pain, weakness in a leg or foot, or any problem controlling your bladder or your bowels, however, your condition should be monitored by a physician.

Eighty percent of persons with sciatica, or leg pain, will eventually recover, with or without treatment. But if you lose control of your bladder as a result of a disc protrusion into your spinal canal, you may need immediate surgery. Most of the time, bladder dysfunction will manifest itself as urinary *retention,* or an inability to empty your bladder. There might also be "saddle anesthesia," or numbness in the portion of your anatomy that fits into a saddle.

It's Probably Only a Strain

If you hurt your back during simple exertion and the pain becomes severe within a day or two, don't panic. Most first-time back pains are the result of simple strain and will usually disappear in a few weeks with no treatment other than rest and moist heat. Except in rare cases where pain is so severe that it's not possible to sleep or visit the toilet, as in the occurrence of a sprain (which is different from a strain) or a ruptured disc, treatment with

SMOKING AND BACK PAIN

According to an article in a 1999 volume of the *American Journal of Public Health,* back pain affects about 17 percent of U.S. workers during the year, costing at least $14 billion in lost workdays! In the same year, *Occupational Medicine* reported that smokers who perform heavy lifting have much more back pain than non-smoking workers. The reason for this is that nicotine supplied by tobacco constricts blood vessels and reduces circulation to tissues, resulting in damage that makes the lower back more susceptible to disease and injury. Researchers at Johns Hopkins University, for example, recently reported that smokers were 25 percent more likely than nonsmokers to develop chronic lower back pain and 84 percent more likely to develop degenerative disc disease in the lumbar spine as a result of diminished blood flow. Reduced circulation can also impede or slow healing, prolonging recovery from injury and increasing chances of reinjury. If you are having back pain, one of the first things you should do is quit smoking. Then, the steps you take to help yourself will be more effective.

painkilling drugs is usually not necessary. If your pain is relieved by lying down and you can sleep all right, chances are you'll be back on your feet in a few days. A strain may result from stretching muscles and tendons. But a sprain, which involves stretching or tearing of ligaments that hold a joint together, is more serious and more painful.

When back pain persists longer than two to four weeks, or if your pain grows progressively worse, with or without leg pain, you should see a doctor for a diagnosis of your problem. In the meantime, there are some basic home treatments that will benefit any kind of back trouble.

We'll begin by discussing ways to relieve back pain. Be sure to read everything in this chapter to see if you can determine what is causing your pain. There are some mechanical-type back problems that persist for months or years, even though they are not serious. You should not be content to endure any kind of chronic back pain month after month without knowing exactly what is causing your pain. You may overlook a serious or progressive disease process (Type O back pain).

Six Steps for Treatment of Simple Back Strain

1. Discontinue activities that seem to increase your back pain.

2. Place an ice pack over the painful area for about twenty minutes every two hours during the first twenty-four to forty-eight hours. This will ease the pain and reduce swelling.

3. Rest in bed only if movement causes severe pain. Try to limit bed rest to two or three days, since prolonged bed rest can lead to weakness or debilitation. Other than for relief of pain, there is no evidence that bed rest speeds recovery from back pain or sciatic-type leg pain.

4. If you need medication for relief of pain, try acetaminophen (Tylenol) first since it has fewer side effects than most medications. If that doesn't help, try an over-the-counter non-steroidal anti-inflammatory medication, such as aspirin, ibuprofen (Advil, Nuprin, Motrin), or naproxen sodium (Naprosyn, Aleve). Remember that prolonged use of acetaminophen can cause liver damage, and use of anti-inflammatory medications for a long period of time (longer than two months) increases risk of liver, kidney, and gastrointestinal problems.

Taking aspirin and other anti-inflammatories with meals will reduce chances of gastrointestinal irritation.

There is also a new class of anti-inflammatory medication called COX-2 inhibitors (Celebrex) now being used in the treatment of arthritis but it must be prescribed by a physician. Be sure to follow the instructions on the bottle for any medications you take—and consult a physician if you have any unusual symptoms or if your pain persists unrelieved. If you are taking blood thinners, cortisone, or some other medication, you should not take anything without the permission of your physician.

5. After two or three days, begin using moist heat over the injured area to speed healing by increasing blood flow. Be guided by the way you feel and use whichever feels best to you. You can also alternate the two.

6. After three or four days, gradually resume your normal activities. Begin with simple walking. Increase the amount of exercise you do over a period of several weeks, including such activities as bicycling or swimming.

Red Flags Indicating Possible Spinal Cancer

If you're over the age of fifty or have a history of cancer, you should always see a physician when you have constant, unrelieved back pain. Unexplained weight loss or back pain that is unrelieved by rest (usually worse at night) or that persists after one month of therapy calls for blood work, a bone scan, or some other test to rule out bone cancer.

Bed Rest for Acute Back Pain

Most persons with low-back pain require bed rest only if they have leg pain that is aggravated by sitting or standing. Occasionally, however, low-back injuries may be so painful that you will be forced to go to bed for relief of symptoms. Simply lying down reduces the load on your lower spine by 75 percent. This reduction in the weight bearing on joints and discs will relieve strain and irritation and allow swelling to subside. Lying down might even allow a bulging disc to move away from a compressed spinal nerve.

Generally, when sudden onset of back pain is so acute that you cannot walk by yourself, it's best to rest in bed a day or two before trying to go to a doctor's office. Chances are you'll feel much better after resting a couple of days. Then, if you still need to see your doctor, getting there won't be such an ordeal. Also, there'll be less chance that you'll get stranded somewhere with a back spasm that's so painful you can't move or get out of your car.

Most of the time, two days of bed rest is enough. More than four days is usually too much. It's much better to get up and move around as much as possible to prevent stiffness in joints and weakness in muscles. Prolonged bed rest can further weaken your spine by allowing inactivity to drain calcium from your vertebrae, especially if you are past middle age. Your bones will retain only the amount of calcium needed to withstand the daily workload. Prolonged bed rest will also slow the circulation of blood through your legs and coronary arteries, contributing to blood clots and heart attacks. So don't lie around any longer than necessary. When back pain is severe, getting in and out of bed to visit the toilet or bathe can be a painful, complicated process. You may not be able to rise to a sitting position as you usually do to get out of bed. You'll have to roll over on your side and push up with your arms while lowering your legs over the side of the bed, taking care not to contract your hip flexors or lift your thighs. Aspirin or acetaminophen might be helpful in reducing painful spasm.

WHEN TO CONSULT YOUR DOCTOR FOR BACK PAIN

Consult your doctor

- if the pain is severe or worsens when lying down;
- if there is unexplained fever over 100 degrees Fahrenheit;
- if the pain is present for more than a month without improvement, occurs at rest, or is worsening;
- if there is unexplained weight loss;
- if there is a history of cancer;
- if there is a history of long-term steroid use, which can weaken the bones and increase susceptibility to fractures;
- if there is recent onset of urinary tract problems, such as pain or burning on urination, increased frequency, or infection;
- if the pain is related to a trauma capable of causing a fracture, such as a high-impact auto accident or a serious fall;

- in the elderly, if there is minor trauma, especially if the person has osteoporosis; or
- if there is severe weakness or numbness in a leg, the genital area, or the buttocks; or if there is a change in the ability to urinate or have a bowel movement. These changes are signs of possible spinal nerve impairment.

Make Sure Your Mattress Is Firm

One of the first requirements for bed rest in treating a painful back is to have a firm bed. If you think your mattress sags too much, place a half-inch–thick sheet of plywood between the mattress and the springs in order to keep the support of your mattress level and uniform. Have the plywood cut to a dimension that's a little smaller than the mattress so that the edges of the plywood won't protrude—and be sure to round the corners.

How Jasper Relieved His Back Pain with a Firm Mattress

Something as simple as a firm mattress will often solve a stubborn back problem. Jasper D. had complained of back trouble for more than a year and had spent thousands of dollars visiting doctors' offices and undergoing physical therapy. "Nothing helped," Jasper recalled, "until I got a new, extra-firm mattress. Since I changed mattresses, my back trouble has practically disappeared!"

A soft, saggy mattress allows the spine to sag, straining joints and ligaments. For your spine to be supported properly, your mattress should be firm enough to keep your spine from sagging but soft enough to mold itself to the curves of your back and hips. When the surface of a mattress feels too hard, you can soften it with a foam rubber covering. Try out a few mattresses, then pick out one that feels best to you.

It is, of course, possible for a mattress or sleeping surface to be too hard. Lying on a hard surface such as a floor will often make back trouble worse by flattening normal curves, since portions of the back will not be supported. A victim of acute back pain who stretches out on the floor for a couple of hours—or overnight—might find it impossible to get up unassisted or without great pain. So if you can barely move, lie on a firm mattress and not on the floor. You can, of course, place your mattress on the floor, but it's usually much easier to get out of a bed than to get up from the floor.

If you have a history of recurring back pain, invest in a good, firm mattress and springs so that you'll be ready for the next attack. If you prefer a water bed, be sure to select a waveless type that contains baffles or compartments to prevent water from moving from one end of the mattress to the other.

Propping Up in Bed

If you want to sit up in bed to read, eat, or watch television while recovering from a back injury, you'll need special support.

Cut a piece of plywood two feet by three feet, cover it with padding, and support it with pillows stacked to hold the board at an angle that supports you comfortably. Keep your knees bent and supported with a pillow.

It's never a good idea to prop up in bed on pillows alone, since this might allow sagging that will place a strain on your spine. If you're fortunate enough to have your own hospital bed, you can simply crank up the upper portion of the bed to get yourself into a well supported, inclined position. You can also crank up the support under your knees.

Relieving Back Pain with Pillows

Many back patients discover that they are most comfortable lying on their side with their knees bent and their hips flexed. A pillow placed between the knees in this position will relieve an uncomfortable pull on the pelvis and hip. Very often, simply lying on your side and pulling your knees up toward your chest will ease back pain and relieve pressure on spinal nerves.

When you lie on your back, it's usually best to place a pillow under your knees so that your knees and your hips are slightly flexed. This produces a little pelvic tilt that allows the lumbar spine to rest in a flattened, relaxed position. If you need more than one pillow to get the support you

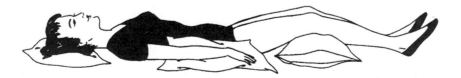

Figure 4-1. Back pain can often be relieved by placing a pillow under the knees to relieve tension on hip flexors and to prevent arching of the lumbar spine.

require under your knees, try rolling up a pillow in a blanket. Or, you can purchase special wedge-shaped pillows that are made to support bent knees. Check with a drugstore that sells hospital supplies.

Lying on your back with your legs flat on the mattress stretches hip-flexor muscles, which in turn pull on the lower lumbar vertebrae. This pull can be very uncomfortable when the lower spine has been injured.

How to Relieve Leg Pain with Sofa Support

Leg pain caused by a pinched spinal nerve in your lower back can sometimes be relieved by lying flat on your back with your lower legs supported horizontally by any padded surface (such as a dining room chair or a stack of sofa cushions) that is higher than your hips.

Sofa traction is especially helpful when back pain is accompanied by leg pain. Lie on the floor on your back and scoot up to the end of the sofa so you can lift your legs over the arm. You can lie this way as long as it feels comfortable.

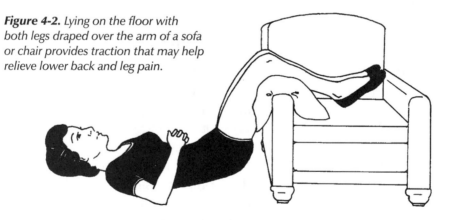

Figure 4-2. Lying on the floor with both legs draped over the arm of a sofa or chair provides traction that may help relieve lower back and leg pain.

How Claire Relieved Her Leg Pain with Sofa Traction

Claire T. discovered on her own that she could relieve her back and leg pain by draping her legs over the arm of a sofa. "I placed a thick pillow over the arm of the sofa so that my hips would be lifted off the floor a little," she explained. "When I lie in this position, I don't have any pain at all."

The pillow Claire placed over the sofa arm was lifting and tilting her pelvis enough to provide the same effect as the pelvic harness used in hospitals to apply low-back traction. Try Claire's sofa traction before investing in the traction apparatus described later in this chapter. Simple knee and hip flexion in a relaxed position will often relieve back pain by reducing tension on the psoas muscles or hip flexors.

Moving Around on Crutches

Most back pain will ease after two or three days of rest. If it becomes apparent that you are unable to walk without assistance after a couple of days, it might be better to try walking with crutches rather than staying in bed and risking muscle weakness. The older you are, the more serious the effects of inactivity or prolonged bed rest, especially if you have osteoporosis (more about this later). A pair of crutches or a walker to support your body weight will often enable you to walk when it wouldn't be possible otherwise.

During the early days of acute back pain, spasms caused by your movement will often buckle your knees, making it difficult to stand. A pair of crutches might help you avoid a fall. Many drugstores rent crutches for temporary use.

Choosing Between Heat and Cold

Moist heat is often used in the treatment of chronic back pain. However, when you have suffered an acute strain or sprain or a muscle injury with discoloration or bruising caused by bleeding in torn muscle fibers, you should always use cold applications during the first forty-eight to seventy-two hours. Otherwise, you may use whichever feels best to you—heat or cold.

To apply moist heat, have someone lay a hot, moist towel over your back. Keep it hot with a hot water bottle, an insulated heating pad, or an infrared lamp.

Never go to sleep using a heating pad. I've seen numerous burns on the backs of people who maintained that the heating pad they slept on was not very hot, but burns can occur when the skin is exposed to long periods of low heat from a pad. Try to limit heat applications to twenty or thirty minutes—and use *moist* heat. You can apply moist heat every two or three hours if you like.

When heat doesn't seem to help, try cold. Crushed ice in a Ziploc bag wrapped in a dry cloth makes a good cold pack. Massaging the back with an ice cube is also often effective for pain relief. Remove the cold when the pain disappears or when the skin becomes numb—usually after fifteen or twenty minutes. Cold may be applied as often as needed to relieve pain.

Constipation Caused by Back Pain

If you have severe back pain, chances are you'll become constipated. Almost without exception, people incapacitated by a back injury will complain of constipation. This is often the result of a reflex mechanism the body uses to protect a painful back from further strain.

Certain prescription painkilling medications may also cause constipation and should not be taken unless absolutely necessary. Strong narcotics can cause nausea or vomiting. More than a few back patients who insisted on taking pain pills because they "couldn't move" had to jump out of bed to vomit after taking the pills. Always try aspirin, acetaminophen, or some other over-the-counter medication before resorting to prescription narcotics or opioids.

Constipation caused by back pain usually corrects itself after three or four days. Eat less to avoid overloading your bowel—and choose your foods carefully. High-fiber fruits and vegetables may be best for guarding against colon impaction. If it appears that constipation is going to be a problem, read the section on constipation in Chapter 2.

When You Need a Back Support

Most back supports are designed to support the lumbar spine by encircling the trunk from the waist down. On rare occasions, a sacroiliac support can be used to support the sacroiliac joints by wrapping a strap tightly around the pelvis.

A back support can be helpful when back pain is so acute that it's difficult to walk or get into and out of a chair. Many drugstores stock a lightweight wrap-around, Velcro-fastening lumbar or lumbosacral support or a sacroiliac support that can be worn safely by anyone. Since uncomplicated low-back injuries usually resolve in two to four weeks, most people will not need a lumbar support. Persons with chronic back pain might benefit from protective support while working. It's not uncommon these days to see employees in the work place wearing such supports outside their clothing.

A heavier, more restricting lumbosacral corset must be prescribed by a physician. Unless you have been chronically incapacitated by severe arthritis, disc herniation, sprain, fracture, or back surgery, it's not likely you'll need to use a heavy corset braced with steel strips—certainly not a rigid brace. There is no evidence to indicate that wearing a lumbar support for periods up to six months will weaken low back muscles. So if a lumbar support feels good to you, it's okay to wear one, especially during periods of exertion. Remember, however, that back supports are useful primarily to relieve and protect a painfully injured back; they may not be helpful in preventing back pain. A study of nine thousand workers, published in a 2000 issue of the *Journal of the American Medical Association,* found no beneficial effects from back belt use among employees who wore belts as a preventative measure, with or without a history of back pain.

Whether you wear a back support or not, you should make a special effort to strengthen your back muscles. Chapter 7 will tell you how to strengthen important abdominal, hip, and back muscles that support your lower spine. If you are recovering from back pain caused by injury, begin with the four special back exercises described at the end of this chapter, when freedom from pain permits.

Disc Problems and the Types of Pain They Cause

Most of the time, your back pain will be the result of simple strain, which might be complicated by arthritis, a structural abnormality, or a joint problem. But when pain, numbness, or tingling radiates down one of your legs, you should suspect disc herniation, especially if you are under sixty years of age.

Since disc cartilage begins to shrink from dehydration after middle age, the older you are, the less likely you'll suffer a disc protrusion. Most often, leg pain in older persons is caused by spinal stenosis or by bony arthritic encroachment upon spinal nerves.

A healthy disc is a thick cartilage cushion that serves as a spacer, a shock absorber, and a ligament between two vertebrae. About one-third of the length of your spinal column is made up of disc cartilage. So there's plenty of opportunity for disc trouble.

When a weak or injured disc ruptures or tears, the soft center portion of the disc sometimes herniates or protrudes from between the vertebrae. This protrusion often hits a spinal nerve, causing symptoms to radiate down one leg. The pain that results is commonly called sciatica. Sometimes a disc will herniate into the end plate of a vertebra, producing a dent, or a Schmorl's node, on the top or bottom surface of the vertebra. End plate injuries or fractures are often painful and difficult to diagnose, but are not as

serious as a disc herniation that protrudes out from between two vertebrae
to pinch a spinal nerve.

When leg pain is increased by
bending forward, a herniated disc is usually indicated. Leg pain that is increased
by bending backward may be due to a
joint spur.

Fortunately, the spinal cord ends at
the level of the second lumbar vertebra.
From there, the spinal nerves pass down,
like hair hanging from a horse's tail
(cauda equina), to exit through openings
(foramina) between the lumbar vertebrae on each side. Protrusion of a lumbar disc into the spinal canal might press
against a few spinal nerves, but it won't
cause total paralysis from the waist down
as some people fear. Since the thick,
heavily loaded lumbar discs are more
subject to herniation than anywhere else
in the spine, nature has reduced the
danger of paralysis by ending the spinal
cord *above* the levels where massive disc
protrusions are common. (Ninety-eight
percent of lumbar disc herniations occur
at the L4–L5 and the L5–S1 level.)

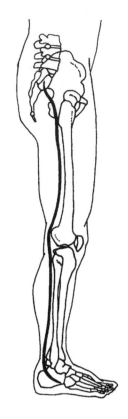

Figure 4-3. *Leg pain caused by disc herniation or spur formation in the lower back most commonly radiates down the sciatic nerve into the leg and foot.*

Remember, however, that a lower lumbar disc protrusion into the spinal
canal can damage nerves supplying muscles that control bladder and bowel
elimination, causing cauda equina syndrome (loss of bladder or bowel control and numbness in the groin).

Most of the time, disc herniation in the lumbar spine will cause weakness or atrophy (shrinkage) in isolated muscles supplied by damaged nerves
in only one portion of one leg. Pain or weakness in both legs may mean that
the spinal canal is involved. MRI or CT scans, myelograms, and other
sophisticated examination methods may be needed to locate spinal nerve
impingement caused by disc herniation or to find a disc fragment or a mass
in the spinal canal.

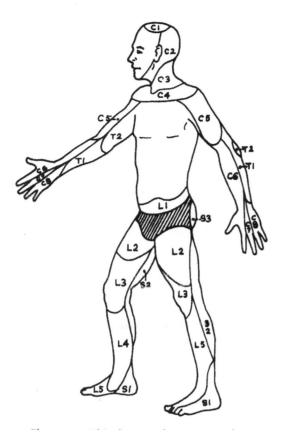

Figure 4-4. *This diagram shows areas where pain, numbness, and other symptoms are commonly felt when spinal nerves in the neck (C) and lower back (L) are pinched or irritated. See page 18 to locate the parts of the spine referred to here.*

How Jonathan Relieved His Leg Pain Using Self-Help

When leg pain is caused by a pinched spinal nerve, it's the back and not the leg that must be treated. In some cases, there may be no back pain at all, only leg pain. Jonathan R. was treating his leg with liniments and hot packs until I convinced him that his leg pain was originating in his back. Once he understood what was causing his leg and foot to hurt, he was able to relieve his pain by using some of the self-help methods described in this chapter.

"Since I can now visualize what's making my leg ache," Jonathan conceded, "I can do more to relieve the symptoms. The home remedies really help! I now know how to avoid irritating the nerve by avoiding postures that make my discs bulge."

See Chapter 9 for tips on how to avoid postures that place pressure on a bad disc.

How to Test for Pinched Nerve Damage

If you begin to experience weakness in the muscles in your thigh, leg, or foot, as in squatting, rising up on your toes, or walking on your heels, you should report these symptoms to your doctor. Those with a history of back and leg pain should be on the lookout for such symptoms since they may indicate nerve damage. Here are a few tests you can do to check for nerve damage:

1. **The knee-jerk test:** Sit on a chair with your legs crossed. Locate the tendon attached to the bottom of your kneecap. Tap this tendon with a flat knife handle.

    Tap both knee tendons and compare the results. If you get a knee jerk on one side and not the other, tell your doctor about this. Weakness or loss of reflex in a knee tendon might indicate disc herniation in the *upper* portion of your lumbar spine.

2. **The ankle-jerk test:** Stand with the shin of one leg supported by a chair seat so that your foot dangles relaxed and unsupported. Have someone tap your ankle tendon with a knife handle. (Be sure to select a dull knife!)

    Check both ankles to see if the response is the same. If you cannot detect a reflex in either ankle, that's okay. But if you have more reflex in one ankle than the other, or if one reflex is absent, that might be an indication of nerve root damage originating at the L5–S1 level at the bottom of your spine. When there are no symptoms, equally undetectable reflexes may not be significant. But when reflexes are not equal, it may indicate nerve damage on one side.

    If the calf muscle on the side with the diminished reflex measures less in circumference than the side with the stronger reflex, you might be developing muscle weakness from nerve damage. You might also have difficulty walking on your toes on the weak side. Your doctor can measure the actual amount of nerve damage with a test called electromyography.

3. **The heel-walk test:** Try walking on your heels, keeping the ball of both feet off the floor. If you are unable to keep one of your feet from dropping flat to the floor, you might have "foot drop," a sign of nerve damage caused by an L4 or L5 disc herniation.

4. **The toe-walk test:** Try walking on your toes, keeping the heels of both feet off the floor. If the heel of one foot falls to the floor and you are unable to walk on your toes, you might have nerve damage due to an L5 disc herniation. If you discover weakness in your foot or leg, you should see a doctor. The doctor will check your ankle reflexes, test the strength of your

legs, measure your calves for muscle shrinkage, and test your skin for loss of sensitivity.

5. **The squat test:** Hold on to a bedpost or other support and squat half way down, first favoring one leg and then the other. If one of your thighs feels weaker than the other, you might have nerve damage from an upper lumbar disc herniation. The knee reflex can be tested by tapping just below the kneecap with the edge of a thin book. Weakness of a thigh muscle and absence of a knee reflex are reasons to consult a doctor.

6. **The straight-leg test:** Sciatica, in which pain radiates from the lower back, through the buttock, and down the back of the thigh into the calf and foot, commonly results from herniation of the L4 or L5 disc (the last two discs at the bottom of the spine), which can compress the L4, L5, and S1 nerve roots. You can test for compression of these spinal nerves by raising the affected leg straight up while lying on your back. If pain on the affected side increases before tension is placed on the hamstrings, usually at a point of less than 60 degrees, that is a good indication that pinching of a nerve root is placing tension on the sciatic nerve.

    You can also do this test by sitting on a table with both hip and knees flexed at 90 degrees and then slowly extending the knee (straightening the leg) on the affected side. If there is a pinched nerve, the pain will force you to lean backward in order to reduce tension on the sciatic nerve.

Discs Don't Slip!

Contrary to popular belief, an intervertebral disc does not "slip." A disc cartilage is made up of dense, tough fibers that are securely attached between two vertebrae. These fibers are normally so strong that they serve as *ligaments* holding the vertebrae together. When a disc is said to "slip," it actually tears or ruptures, which may allow herniation or protrusion of the soft center of the disc.

There is no manipulation that will replace a "slipped disc." Sometimes, however, manipulation performed by a chiropractor, an osteopath, or a physical therapist will relieve symptoms by stretching tight muscles and mobilizing stiff joints. Improper or excessive manipulation can, of course, worsen the symptoms of a disc protrusion, especially when the protrusion is massive enough to encroach upon a spinal nerve. So while manipulation will sometimes do more harm than good in the treatment of a freshly herniated disc, traction or spinal stretching is always safe, provided it can be applied without pain, even if it doesn't always help.

Ruptured Discs Always Degenerate

Over a period of several years, a ruptured or herniated disc will degenerate, narrowing the disc space and causing the vertebrae to move too close together. This results in slipping or overriding of vertebral joints or facets, causing arthritic stiffness and binding. When this happens, manipulation might be more effective than traction in relieving symptoms.

SUGGESTION: DON'T BE IN A HURRY FOR BACK SURGERY!

■ If you suddenly develop symptoms of a lumbar disc herniation, you won't need emergency surgery unless you have cauda equina syndrome (loss of bladder or bowel control and numbness in the groin or "saddle area"), which is rare. It takes twelve to sixteen weeks for a herniated disc to heal, and 85 to 90 percent can be treated without surgery. Even when there is sciatic-type leg pain (pinched nerve), 80 percent eventually recover. Remember that a herniated disc, which is tissue composed largely of water, will dehydrate and shrink over a period of time, thus relieving irritating pressure on nerves. If no nerve damage is taking place, as determined by periodic examination by a physician, you can postpone surgery as long as you can tolerate the pain.

■ When symptoms worsen despite time and conservative treatment and there is progressive nerve damage taking place, your doctor might advise you not to wait longer than a few months to have back surgery if there is a direct correlation between MRI findings and your symptoms. For example, if it is confirmed that you have a massive L5 disc herniation with weakness in corresponding foot structures, you might risk development of a permanent "foot flop" if you postpone surgery too long. It's your choice and your risk.

Buying Time with Traction

Traction is not as effective on the lower back as it is on the neck. It might even aggravate acute back pain that is caused by a strain or a sprain. Very few doctors now recommend spinal traction as a treatment for back pain caused by a ruptured disc. It might be worth trying spinal traction at home, however, when you have leg pain that is not relieved by lying down. If you have chronic or recurring back pain due to disc degeneration, arthritis, facet misalignment, or some other mechanical problem, there's a good chance that low-back stretching or traction will relax muscles and relieve pressure on sensitive spinal joints. The pelvic tilt provided by properly applied traction may even widen the openings (foramina) between the lower lumbar vertebrae enough to relieve chronic leg pain caused by nerve root irritation.

How Jason D. and Grace C. Relieve Pain with Self-Help

Jason D. suffers from recurring back pain caused by disc degeneration and facet joint displacement. "When I have back pain after working in my yard," Jason explained, "I hook up my traction and stretch my back with 30 or 40 pounds for a few minutes. This always results in some degree of immediate relief from the pain."

Grace C. prefers manipulation for relief of pain caused by a degenerated disc. When she is unable to visit my office, she uses some of the home manipulation techniques described in Chapter 5. "Most of the time," she says, "I can relieve my back pain by stretching and loosening my spine at home."

If low-back traction does relieve back or leg pain, the traction should be used as much and as often as possible. If you have a herniated disc, anything you can do to relieve pain will put time on your side. Remember that if you allow enough time for a ruptured or herniated disc to degenerate, your chances of needing surgery will be reduced. Once a disc is fully degenerated, there is not enough cartilage left to bulge out against a nerve and nothing left to remove surgically. The arthritis that results from overriding of joint facets is something you can live with and that can be relieved with traction at home.

Unlike a simple strain that might resolve in a week or two, it may take several weeks for the pain of a ruptured disc to subside. You should allow yourself weeks and months for recovery. Surgery won't be indicated unless you have muscle weakness, an absent reflex (radiculopathy), and other symptoms of nerve damage caused by impingement of a spinal nerve.

Usually, a ruptured disc is simply a tear in the disc cartilage without nerve root involvement. When leg pain is present, this usually means that the disc has herniated or protruded out against a spinal nerve. You won't need surgery for a ruptured disc unless it herniates and produces nerve symptoms.

If you have a ruptured disc and are overweight, you should begin by reducing your body weight to lessen the chances of herniation (see Chapter 6). Taking a few hundred milligrams of vitamin C daily might also help by strengthening disc cartilage. Remember, however, that doses larger than 200 milligrams are excreted and not used by the body, and there is no evidence that larger doses might be beneficial.

Once a disc ruptures, whether it herniates or not, it leaves a weakened, unstable spinal joint that might result in chronic or recurring back pain. Self-help in a back-care program then becomes a life-long necessity.

How to Use Traction at Home to Relieve Back and Leg Pain

There are several ways to stretch your back at home. You can use a special harness to stretch your back in bed, or you can use some other method that does not involve the use of pulleys. You might want to try them all to see which works best for you.

Pelvic Harness Traction

Traction applied with a pulley and a harness fastened around the pelvis is the most popular method of stretching the lower back. A weight is attached to the end of a cord that runs from the harness and over a pulley that is fastened to the foot of the bed. (Usually, cords from each side of the harness attach to a spreader bar, from which a single cord passes over a single pulley.)

A surgical supply store will sell or rent you a pulley apparatus that can be hung over a footboard or clamped to a mattress. Some enterprising patients build their own traction equipment after seeing traction demonstrated.

The traction cord should pull uphill about 25 degrees so that the pelvis is lifted slightly, or tilted upward. A pillow or roll placed under the knees will help maintain a comfortable pelvic tilt, thus enhancing the traction. A couple of bricks placed under each foot post of the bed will also help make the traction more effective by adding the effect of countergravity.

VITAMIN C ESSENTIAL FOR STRONG DISCS

Since vitamin C is essential for building and repairing collagen in disc fibers, an effort should be made to eat five servings of vitamin C–rich fruits and vegetables each day, such as oranges, strawberries, Brussels sprouts, or broccoli. In the absence of a good diet, a 200-milligram vitamin C supplement might be beneficial.

RICH SOURCES OF VITAMIN C

Food	Serving size	Mg. of vitamin C
Brussels sprouts	½ cup	68
Strawberries	¾ cup	66
Orange	1	66
Orange juice	½ cup	60
Broccoli	½ cup	52
Grapefruit juice	½ cup	48
White grapefruit	½	44
Pink grapefruit	½	44
Collard greens	½ cup	44
Mustard greens	½ cup	34
Cauliflower	½ cup	33
Cantaloupe	¼	32
Tangerine	1	27
Cabbage	½ cup	24
Cooked tomatoes	½ cup	21
Tomato juice	½ cup	20

The recommended daily allowance for vitamin C is 90 milligrams for men and 75 milligrams for women. Smokers may need an additional 35 milligrams daily.

There is evidence to indicate that the body cannot absorb more than 100 milligrams of vitamin C a day and that blood is saturated at 200 milligrams. Any amount over 200 milligrams is therefore excreted through the kidneys. For this reason, vitamin C supplements taken to repair and improve production of collagen need not exceed 200 milligrams.

4

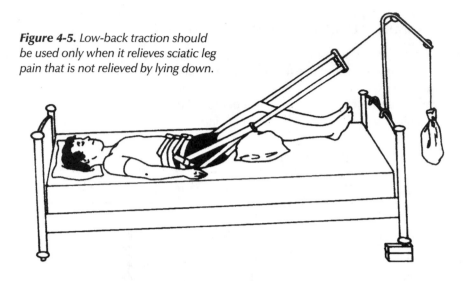

Figure 4-5. Low-back traction should be used only when it relieves sciatic leg pain that is not relieved by lying down.

Selecting a Weight for Pelvic Traction

Begin your traction by using a 15- or 20-pound weight for half an hour or longer. If no ill effects occur, gradually work up to 30 or 40 pounds. Select a weight that feels best for you; that is, a weight that seems to relieve your back or leg pain.

Traction should never be painful. Discontinue it if it cannot be adjusted to relieve your symptoms. Remember that traction is used primarily to relieve back or leg pain that is not eased by lying down. If you do not have any pain while lying down, simple bed rest may be adequate and you may not need traction. Be guided by the way you feel. If traction feels good, use it; if it causes pain, don't use it.

How to Stretch Your Spine Without a Pulley

The most simple way to stretch your spine is to suspend your body and let gravity do the rest.

Chair traction: Place two sturdy chairs back-to-back. Stand between the chairs and place both hands on top of the chair backs. Support your weight with straight arms and let your body relax from the waist down. Leave your feet resting on the floor, but keep your legs relaxed so that they don't support any weight. Suspend your weight for several seconds or until your arms become fatigued.

Door traction: Stand a foot away from an open door. Then lean into the door and grasp the top of the door with both hands. Let your knees bend and your body sag so that you are suspending your weight with your arms. Let your feet rest on the floor but don't support any weight with your legs.

With a little practice, you should be able to relax enough to feel your spine stretch from the pull of your body weight.

How Dayton Used an Open Door to Relieve Back and Leg Pain

Dayton B. was a busy accountant who spent many hours each day sitting at his desk. Back and leg pain that had been diagnosed as a "bulging disc" was being aggravated by sitting, making his day long and miserable.

"I have to get up frequently and walk around to relieve the pain," Dayton complained. "It's getting more difficult to sit for more than an hour or two."

I showed Dayton how to stretch his spine several different ways in his office. He tried them all and decided that the door method was best for him. "Hanging from the door relieves my back and leg pain," he reported. "If I hang from the door several times a day, I can work a full day without too much difficulty."

Be Cautious with Inversion Traction

Not too many years ago, some people were using free-hanging inversion boots to stretch their spines. The body was suspended upside down from boots that were attached to an overhead bar or doorframe.

Since blood pressure increases tremendously when the body is suspended upside down, I do not recommend free-hanging inversion boots. The risk of unconsciousness or eye hemorrhage is too great to consider such treatment.

If you're going to use an inversion apparatus to stretch your spine, however, it would be better to lie on a tilting frame that you can control so that you can tilt the frame to an angle that's comfortable for you. With your feet secured at the high end of the frame, an angle from 45 to 75 degrees should be enough to stretch your spine.

Simply lying on a slanted board with your feet anchored at the high end of the board is also a fairly effective way to stretch your spine.

Some therapists use gravity traction, in which the patient is strapped at chest level to a tilting table and then suspended upright at an angle of 60 or

70 degrees. This allows gravity and the weight of the lower body to stretch the lumbar spine. This method of gravity traction is much safer than inversion traction, since there is no danger of rupturing a blood vessel in the eye or around the brain. Gravity traction might also be more effective than traction applied while lying in bed.

Dealing with Structural Abnormalities

When back trouble persists or recurs frequently, it is often the result of a structural abnormality in the lower spine. Deformities affecting the shape of the vertebrae or the way the joints fit together may place a strain on ligaments or cause chronic irritation of facets or joint surfaces. An overexertion or a jolt on an abnormal joint can result in acute pain that may last for several days and then disappear, recurring weeks or months later when the affected joints are again banged together or strained.

The most common types of lower back problems I see in my practice, other than those caused by strains and sprains, are those involving arthritis, curvatures, and lumbosacral (located at the very bottom of the spine) joint deformities.

You'll learn how to recognize and care for the various types of spinal arthritis when you read Chapter 8.

How Spinal Curvatures Cause Back Pain

Very few people have a perfectly straight spine. It's not uncommon for one leg to be a little shorter than the other, lowering the pelvis enough on one side to cause the spine to curve from side to side. Structural asymmetry or uneven joints in the lower part of the spine (detected only by X-ray exam) can also result in a spinal curvature.

Most structural (permanent) curvatures are simply compensatory curves developed by the body to counteract imbalances. It's not uncommon, for example, for the thoracic spine to curve toward the arm you use most. My old edition of *Gray's Anatomy* noted that the thoracic spine has a slight lateral curvature, with the curve going to the right in right-handed persons and to the left in left-handed persons. More than one person has undergone spinal manipulation in an attempt to "correct" this curve! But natural asymmetry in spinal joints may cause slight curvatures that are needed to balance stresses on the vertebral column.

Most of us have some abnormal curves in our spine. When these curves do not cause trouble, they are not a cause for alarm. When a curvature exceeds certain limits, however, strain placed on joints, ligaments, and discs can cause problems.

Generally, if your back is not bothering you and you cannot detect any obvious imbalance when you see your image in a mirror, it's not likely that you have enough of a curvature to be a problem. So don't be frightened by the pessimistic reports of practitioners who conduct "postural checks" in malls while passing out their business cards.

Note: Exaggerated normal curves, such as sway back or the hump back of poor posture, can be a cause of back pain. These types of curves are discussed in Chapter 9. In this chapter, we're considering only abnormal side-to-side curves, such as the S-shaped scoliosis curvature.

A Mirror Test for Scoliosis

You can often detect an S-shaped spinal curvature simply by analyzing your posture in a mirror. If one shoulder is higher than the other and one arm hangs farther away from your body on one side than on the other, or if one hip seems to be higher than the other, causing your pants legs to hang unevenly, chances are you have some curvature in your spine. If you're also having back trouble, you might have enough of a curvature to place uneven pressure on spinal joints. This can lead to the development of arthritis in chronically irritated joints, requiring occasional treatment for relief of symptoms.

How to Examine the Spine for Scoliosis

The best way to test for the presence of a curvature or scoliosis in the spine is to

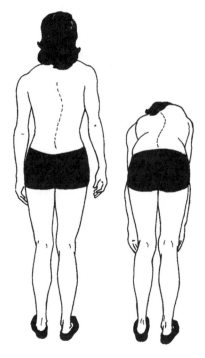

Figure 4-6. *When scoliosis is present, a hump is apparent on one side of the back when you bend forward.*

have someone observe the changes that occur in your back while you are bending forward.

Have the person examining you sit behind you. Then, slowly bend over with your head down and both arms hanging loosely.

If a hump appears on one side of the surface of the upper back during the first half of bending, this usually means that the spine is rotated or curved to that side enough to cause the ribs to protrude back on the convex side of the curvature.

If muscles bulge on the opposite side of the spine as you continue to bend forward, this means that there is an S-shaped curvature, or scoliosis, that might be pronounced enough to be a problem. When this curvature is caused by one leg being shorter than the other, a heel lift might help.

THE ABCs OF SCOLIOSIS

- Scoliosis, in which two side-to-side curves form an "S" shape, is not often a cause of back pain in adults when the curves measure less than 20 degrees.

- Scoliosis in an adult cannot be corrected but can be treated for symptomatic relief.

- Idiopathic scoliosis (scoliosis for which the cause is not known) in children may require bracing or surgery if the curvature progresses 20 degrees.

- Most structural forms of scoliosis reach a maximum level of deformity by age sixteen, but a progressive idiopathic scoliosis that is not halted during childhood may progress past 60 degrees, causing crippling deformity and life-threatening compression of vital organs.

- Spinal curvatures in children between the ages of six and sixteen should always be brought to the attention of an orthopedic specialist. Close observation may be required to determine if there is a progressive idiopathic scoliosis that might require bracing or surgery.

Stretching your spine at home, as recommended earlier in this chapter, might relieve some of the symptoms resulting from a curvature. The exercises described in Chapter 7 should be done regularly to build the muscle support you need to keep your curving spine from sagging under the pull of gravity.

Good posture is also important. It's essential that you do all you can to improve your posture when sitting, standing, or lying down, as recommended in Chapter 9.

In many cases, the techniques I recommend for loosening and aligning the spine at home (Chapter 5) will relieve symptoms caused by a stiff spine or jammed joints.

Note: If you're over the age of eighteen, don't be alarmed if your doctor tells you that you have a slight scoliosis. Most scoliotic curvatures in adults are not progressive and will not be a problem unless they are severe enough to place a strain on joints and ligaments. A structural scoliosis is not correctable and cannot be "straightened out." So don't be persuaded to undergo long courses of spinal manipulation to "correct your alignment."

Children between the ages of six to sixteen with any type of curvature, particularly scoliosis, should be kept under the observation of an orthopedic specialist. Progression of a scoliosis beyond 20 degrees may be an indication of a possible need for surgery.

How Arty T. Used Home Remedies to Relieve Pain Caused by a Spinal Curvature

Arty, a sixty-eight-year-old chemist, started having chronic backache for the first time in his life a few years after his retirement. X-ray examination revealed a large spur formation on the concave side of a spinal curvature.

After trying various forms of treatment, Arty concluded that spinal stretching provided the most relief from symptoms. "When I overdo it and develop a backache," he observed, "I can usually get relief by using moist heat and stretching my spine at home."

Try a variety of home treatments before undergoing a long course of therapy in a doctor's office. You might get better results as well as save yourself some money.

Correcting Curvatures with a Shoe Lift

Curvatures caused by an uneven leg length can sometimes be improved by placing a lift in the shoe on the side with the short leg. This must be done under the supervision of a chiropractor or an orthopedist, however; improper or unnecessary use of a shoe lift might worsen symptoms or create new problems. Without special examination or measuring procedures, it's often difficult to be sure which leg is short, since a scoliosis might create the illusion that one hip is higher than the other.

Remember that scoliosis can occur even when both leg lengths are perfectly equal. So don't attempt to use a heel lift or a shoe lift based on what you see in a mirror.

Generally, the older you are, the less helpful a shoe lift will be, since bony changes in your vertebrae might make it impossible to alter the curves of your spine. For most of us, a shoe lift would not be helpful. If you have back pain that you feel might be caused by uneven leg length, and wearing a heel lift seems to help, use one. It's not a good idea, however, to use a heel lift greater than one-quarter of an inch in height. A congenital leg deficiency of less than two centimeters (about three-quarters of an inch) is not believed to be a significant factor in the production of back pain. It's never a good idea to attempt correction of more than one-half of a measured structural leg deficiency in an adult. Leg length should be carefully measured before adding a shoe lift.

How to Handle Common Low-Back Joint Deformities

Even when the spine is perfectly straight and has normal curves, abnormalities in the bones and joints of the lower spine can be a cause of backache. In fact, lumbosacral joint deformities (at the base of the spine) are a common cause of chronic backache.

Lumbosacral facets (joints) are sometimes improperly developed or tilted the wrong way, causing them to jam or become overloaded (facet syndrome). Occasionally, the bony bridge connecting two interlocking joints may be absent or broken apart (spondylolysis), allowing one vertebra to slip forward over the vertebra below (spondylolisthesis). This happens most often to the fifth lumbar vertebra, which slips on the downhill slope of the spine's supporting foundation (the sacrum). This might cause a visible notch or "step" at the bottom of the spine, just above the dimples on the back of the pelvis.

Monitoring Spondylolisthesis

There are two types of spondylolisthesis. One is the result of a degenerative process that allows the uppermost vertebra to slip forward a little. This condition never requires surgery, since the joints locking the vertebrae together remain intact.

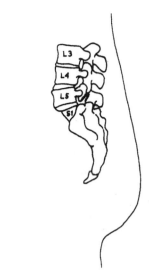

Figure 4-7.
Spondylolisthesis, or forward slipping of a vertebra, most commonly occurs in the lumbosacral area of the spine.

The other type of spondylolisthesis is more serious and sometimes requires surgery. In true spondylolisthesis, there is a congenital defect in the interlocking joints, which allows the locking structures to separate, as in a fracture. When this happens, the vertebra above is held in place only by disc cartilage and ligaments. As you grow older and the disc cartilage degenerates, the vertebra may begin slipping forward more rapidly, held in place only by the restraining ligaments. This type of spondylolisthesis must be kept under observation by X ray (if the condition is causing back or leg pain) to determine if there is enough progressive slipping to warrant surgical fusion. When a spondylolisthesis is a grade 1 or 2, it might not be much of a problem. If it progresses to a grade 3 or 4, however, which is quite rare, there may be a real problem, requiring the attention of an orthopedic surgeon.

Fortunately, most persons who have a spondylolisthesis get along quite well, with only chronic or recurring backache. A lumbar support, moist heat, the spinal stretching techniques described in this chapter, or simply pulling the knees up to the chest while lying down may relieve symptoms.

How Myra B.'s "Nervous Backache" Was Caused by Spondylolysis

Twenty-year-old Myra B. had been working at her new job as a bank teller for only a few months when she began to complain of severe backache. When she started missing time at work, her employer accused her of goofing off. Her family physician checked to be certain there was no infection in the kidneys, then suggested that her backache was caused by "nerves."

An X-ray examination revealed that Myra was actually suffering from spondylolysis that had not yet started to cause slipping of the involved vertebra. "I'm sure glad to know that my backache is not all in my head," she confessed with relief.

I recommended a temporary lumbosacral support for Myra and prescribed exercises such as those described in Chapter 7. "I'm doing much better now," she reported a few weeks later. "My boss is more sympathetic and is no longer threatening to fire me."

Of course, stress can cause backache, but such a diagnosis should not be made until structural problems have been ruled out.

Transitional Vertebrae: Mixed-Up Joints

A transitional vertebra is a congenital deformity in which the last vertebra in the spine has characteristics of the lumbar spine above and the supporting sacral base below. The result is a vertebra that has an excessive or abnormal bony attachment to both portions of the spine. Often, there may be one lumbar vertebra too many or one too few. In either case, abnormal bony development may cause recurring backache that is not serious and that can often be relieved by rest and other simple home treatments.

Unlike spondylolisthesis, which may require that the loose, slipping vertebra be anchored surgically to protect important spinal nerves, a transitional vertebra is usually structurally secure and won't slip out of alignment. It may, however, result in localized arthritis or joint pain from jamming or irritation of abnormal bony surfaces. Your doctor might diagnose the problem as a lumbarized first sacral segment or a sacralized fifth lumbar vertebra, which is the same as a transitional vertebra.

Most of the time, a transitional vertebra does not present a serious problem. But if you have such a vertebra, you should avoid placing excessive strain or leverage on your lower back in order to avoid injuring abnormal joints.

How Knowing the Cause Helped Leona B. Handle Her Back Pain

Leona B. was relieved to learn that her chronic backache was being caused by a transitional vertebra. "Now that I know what my problem is," she said, "I can live with the symptoms. Besides, from what I now know about my back, I'll be able to protect it better and treat it better at home."

Moving Away from Back Pain

You already know that the pain of a ruptured disc may be aggravated by bending forward, while joint pain might be aggravated by bending backward. Low-back structural deformities might be painful with movement in any direction. When there is a transitional vertebra, which is often abnormally attached on one side, pain might be more evident when bending to one side.

If you have a "kissing spine," leaning backward might trigger a backache. When the spinous processes (the bony projections or bumps in the center of the spine) are too close together in the lower portion of the spine, bending backward causes them to "kiss" or pinch together, irritating bony surfaces. Working with your arms overhead, as in painting a ceiling, might cause severe back pain if you have a kissing spine.

Obviously, when movement in a certain direction is painful, you should avoid moving in that direction. You might, in fact, be able to relieve the pain by moving or bending in the *opposite* direction. Be guided by the way you feel. Don't do any exercise that causes pain. Avoid postures or positions that cause discomfort. *If it hurts, don't do it!*

Since most back pains originate in the *joints* of the spine, which are on the back side of the spine, you can often relieve back pain simply by pulling your knees up toward your chest or resting your legs upon a chair seat or over the arm of a sofa (see the illustration on page 82). The pelvic tilt induced by many of the postural exercises recommended for the alleviation of back pain are designed to relieve pressure on painful spinal joints.

Any of the various home treatments described in this chapter will provide some symptomatic relief for almost any Type M, or mechanical, back problems. All of these treatments are safe; if one doesn't help, try another.

Prevention and Treatment for Osteoporosis (Brittle Vertebrae)

We have all seen older ladies—and a few old men—with a "dowager's hump," a slumping of the upper spine. "My mother had such a hump," recalled one gray-haired lady, "and now I have one. I guess I inherited it from her."

When the spine suddenly begins to slump after middle age, it's not likely that the cause is inherited. If you do not now have a hump on your back, it's unlikely that you'll have one if you do what you should to *prevent* one from developing.

Spinal humps that develop late in life, especially in females after menopause, are almost always caused by osteoporosis, a thinning of bones (loss of density) from calcium deficiency. In most cases, the lack of adequate calcium intake that began long before menopause has already reduced bone density considerably. Then, at menopause, when the estrogen level drops, the bones begin to lose calcium more rapidly, making the vertebrae porous, brittle, and weak. This loss of bone may not be evident on X-ray examination, however, until the loss is 30 percent or greater. This means that when symptoms develop and the hump begins to appear, the disease has been developing for many years. When a vertebral body collapses, loss of support on the front side of the spine allows the portion of the spine above to tilt forward, forming a hump in the back. As more vertebrae collapse, the worse the hump becomes.

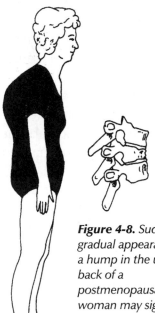

Figure 4-8. *Sudden or gradual appearance of a hump in the upper back of a postmenopausal woman may signal the presence of a collapsed vertebra caused by advanced osteoporosis.*

Low calcium and hormonal levels combined with poor eating habits and lack of exercise may cause such rapid calcium loss that the weakened bones of the spine begin to collapse under the pressure of body weight. This usually becomes evident first in the lower or middle thoracic area (between the shoulder blades) where the natural curve of the spine places compression on the vertebrae. As the spine begins to slump, the compression increases, literally crushing some of the vertebrae.

In osteoporosis, the vertebrae are porous and brittle as a result of inadequate calcium in the bone. In osteomalacia, the vertebrae have normal density but are soft because of a deficiency in the minerals and vitamin D needed to harden the bone. Fortunately, you can prevent both of these diseases with one treatment program.

Back-Weakening Osteoporosis Can Be Prevented!

Most of the time, slumping of the spine and compression of the vertebrae can be prevented with proper attention to diet, exercise, and posture in early and middle years. Once osteoporosis develops and the vertebrae become compressed or crushed, the damaged vertebrae can never be restored to their original strength, and compression results in deformity and shortened height.

Pain and deformity caused by the collapse of osteoporotic vertebrae can be minimized with a new procedure called percutaneous vertebroplasty. In this procedure, sterile liquid cement is injected into the fractured vertebral bodies, filling holes and crevasses to strengthen the vertebrae and prevent further collapse. When a balloon is used to expand the collapsed vertebrae before the cement is injected, the procedure is called kyphoplasty.

In order to keep osteoporosis under control and prevent a spinal hump from getting worse, you must increase your intake of calcium and other minerals and vitamins by eating properly and taking supplements. You should also do special exercises to strengthen the muscles supporting your spine. Exercise will strengthen your vertebrae, since bones retain or absorb more calcium when they are subjected to stress. Your bones will, in fact, lose calcium and grow weaker if you are totally inactive, even if you are getting adequate calcium in your diet. So if you want to keep your bones strong, you must exercise regularly and eat properly.

Older people who are totally inactive may develop such weak bones that a hip will fracture spontaneously while they are walking, or a vertebra could collapse while they are just sitting or coughing. It's not uncommon for people suffering from osteoporosis to fracture ribs while reaching over the back of a car seat.

Diet in the Treatment and Prevention of Osteoporosis

A deficiency of calcium in the diet is, in my opinion, probably the biggest factor in the development of osteoporosis. Even when the diet supplies adequate calcium, however, certain other dietary imbalances can create a calcium deficiency.

Ideally, your diet should supply equal amounts of calcium and phosphorus—or a little more calcium than phosphorus. Excessive consumption of phosphorus-rich meats (fish, fowl, or red meat) can supply such an excessive amount of phosphorus that calcium is actually drained from the body. (When excess phosphorus is eliminated by the kidneys, some calcium is eliminated, too.) For this reason, cola drinks, which are high in phosphorus, should be consumed sparingly.

Too much salt (sodium) in your diet can also drain calcium from your body. As in the case of excess phosphorus, calcium is eliminated by your kidneys along with excess sodium. Every time you salt a big steak, the excess phosphorus and sodium might cause you to lose a little calcium. A couple of hamburgers and a cola is an anti-calcium meal and should not be eaten regularly.

Obviously, it's important to eat a variety of fresh, natural foods and a low-salt, balanced diet that includes all the major nutritional groups. This will assure an adequate intake of calcium without an imbalance in nutrients. You'll learn how to balance your diet when you read Chapter 6.

Getting Adequate Vertebrae-Building Calcium from Food

Dairy products, such as milk, yogurt, and cheese, are the best sources of calcium. Dark green, leafy vegetables, such as spinach, collards, and mustard greens, also contain calcium, but in a form not easily absorbed. Sardines and canned salmon (with bones) are good sources of calcium. A quart of milk or its equivalent in milk products supplies a little more than 1,000 milligrams of calcium (the recommended daily allowance) with a little less than 1,000 milligrams of phosphorus—which is a good ratio of calcium to phosphorus.

It's difficult to get adequate calcium without including milk products in the diet. Unfortunately, many adults do not have the digestive enzyme needed to digest lactose, or milk sugar, resulting in flatulence and other digestive disturbances. When milk is fermented to form cheese, yogurt, or buttermilk, however, the lactose is converted to lactic acid by bacterial activity, making the milk easier to digest. So if you can't tolerate fresh milk, try a fermented milk product. You can also take a tablet containing a lactase enzyme when you drink milk. Such tablets are available in any drugstore, and most supermarkets now sell milk that contains a lactase additive.

After menopause, or when it has been established that you have osteoporosis, your need for calcium increases. You should try to make sure that a combination of diet and supplements supplies at least 1,500 milligrams of calcium a day. If you are elderly, you may have to take betaine hydrochloride (acid) tablets (available in drugstores and health food stores, often in combination with digestive enzymes) with meals (along with a calcium supplement), to assure greater absorption of calcium. Taking vitamin C, or ascorbic acid, with meals will also increase absorption of calcium.

FOOD SOURCES OF CALCIUM

Milk and milk products are the best sources of calcium. The calcium in plant foods is not readily absorbed. A glass of milk, for example, contains 315 milligrams of calcium, of which 101 milligrams are absorbed. A serving of spinach, on the other hand, contains 129 milligrams of calcium, and only 7 milligrams are absorbable.

It's important to eat a variety of foods from all the basic food groups each day in order to meet daily nutritional requirements for vitamins and minerals.

Remember that taking sodium bicarbonate and other calcium-free antacids will decrease absorption of calcium. Aluminum-containing antacids will result in excretion of calcium. A calcium-containing antacid such as TUMS is a good source of calcium (two tablets containing 400 milligrams of elemental calcium), but I usually recommend calcium carbonate (one tablet, 600 milligrams of elemental calcium) with vitamin D, which is cheaper and does not contain sugar or flavoring. Most American women consume only about 450 milligrams of calcium daily from foods. Much of this is not absorbed when there is a deficiency of stomach acid, especially in elderly women.

Supplementing the Diet with Calcium Pills

When osteoporosis becomes advanced, it may not be possible to get adequate calcium from the average diet. It might be necessary to supplement a "calcium-rich" diet with several hundred milligrams of calcium daily to assure an intake of at least 1,500 milligrams.

There are many kinds of calcium supplements on the market. Some are too low in calcium, however, and some may cause digestive disturbances or interfere with the elimination of waste from the body. If you are intolerant to lactose (milk sugar), for example, it might be best to avoid calcium lactate. Calcium carbonate (a common ingredient of antacids) can cause constipation in some people.

You may have to experiment with the various types of calcium to find one that agrees with you. Some people prefer oyster shell calcium, bone meal, or dolomite. Both bone meal and dolomite, however, have been accused of sometimes being contaminated with such toxic metals as lead.

Calcium citrate or calcium ascorbate, which is calcium combined with a form of vitamin C, provides an easily absorbed form of calcium. Your doctor might prescribe a calcium supplement designed especially for you. Oyster shell calcium may provide as much as 500 milligrams of calcium in one tablet. Most calcium carbonate supplements, the most commonly prescribed form of calcium, provide 600 milligrams of calcium in a single tablet.

CALCIUM REQUIREMENTS FOR MEN AND WOMEN

	Age	Dosage (Milligrams)
Men	25–65	1,000
	65+	1,500
Women	25–50	1,000
	(Pregnant or nursing)	1,500
	65+ (taking estrogen)	1,000
	65+ (not taking estrogen)	1,500

Note: 400 to 800 International Units of vitamin D are required daily to maintain normal levels of calcium in the blood.

Taking more than 600 milligrams of calcium at one time may result in the excretion of the calcium through the kidneys, so taking one supplement at night and one in the morning may work best. The National Academy of Sciences has advised that consumption of more than 2,500 milligrams of calcium daily may cause kidney stones or damage the kidneys.

Figuring Calcium Intake

Calcium combined with other substances, such as gluconate, carbonate, or lactate in tablet form, is not all calcium. Calcium carbonate usually supplies the greatest amount of calcium per tablet. One tablet that contains 1,000 milligrams of calcium carbonate, for example, may supply 400 milligrams of calcium, while 1,000 milligrams of calcium lactate may contain only 130 milligrams of calcium. A tablet containing 1,000 milligrams of calcium gluconate might supply only 10 milligrams of calcium, which is hardly worthwhile for a person with osteoporosis. One teaspoon of bone meal, on the other hand, contains 120 milligrams of calcium, while one teaspoon of dolomite (calcium carbonate with magnesium) contains 1,180 milligrams of calcium. Be sure to read calcium supplement labels carefully to determine how much "elemental calcium" each tablet contains.

Remember, too, that you need vitamin D to absorb and utilize calcium and to prevent osteomalacia as well as osteoporosis. Try to supplement your diet with at least 400 units of vitamin D daily, preferably in combination with calcium or in milk. However, you should never take more than 1,000 units of vitamin D in one day. While you need a certain amount to maintain a proper level of calcium in your blood, too much vitamin D can withdraw calcium from your bones and deposit it in your soft tissues. Worst of all, vitamin D can be toxic when an excessive amount is stored in the body.

FOOD SOURCES OF BONE-BUILDING CALCIUM

Dairy Products	mg
Yogurt, nonfat plain (1 cup)	488
Milk, skim (1 cup)	301
Milk, whole (1 cup)	290
Cheese (1 oz)*	195–335
Yogurt, frozen vanilla (1 cup)	206
Fish and Shellfish (3 oz)	
Atlantic sardines, with bones, canned	324
Pink salmon, with bones, canned	181
Blue crab	85
Fruits and Vegetables	
Figs, dried (5)	135
Collard greens (1/2 cup, cooked)	113
Bok choy (1/2 cup, cooked)	79
Orange (1 medium)	61
Mustard greens (1/2 cup, cooked)	52
Butternut squash (1/2 cup, cooked)	50
Kale (1/2 cup, cooked)	47
Grains	
Amaranth (1/2 cup)	149
English muffin (1)	101

Grains (cont'd)

Bagel (1)	50
Bread, whole wheat (2 slices)	40

Legumes

Tofu, with calcium sulfate (1/2 cup, cooked)	434
Black-eyed peas (1/2 cup, cooked)	95
Almonds (1/4 cup)	90
Navy beans (1/2 cup, cooked)	64
Great northern beans (1/2 cup, cooked)	60

Syrup

Blackstrap molasses (1 tablespoon)	176

*The harder the cheese, the higher the calcium content

In especially difficult cases of osteoporosis, you should consult an orthopedic specialist for advice on the use of chemicals or drugs that might help increase bone density. Doctors sometimes prescribe estrogen along with calcium to assure greater retention of calcium. Fluorides, alendronate (Fosamax), etidronate, and other drugs might be prescribed to harden bones. Special hormones, such as calcitonin, might be injected into the body to slow bone loss.

No matter what kind of drugs or supplements you take, you must also eat a good, balanced diet. You need vitamin C, zinc, magnesium, phosphorus, protein, and other nutrients, as well as calcium and vitamin D, to build the framework your body needs for the construction of strong, dense bones.

Note: Regular use of mineral oil laxatives will wash fat-soluble vitamin D out of your intestinal tract, contributing to the development of both osteoporosis and osteomalacia. Some diet foods may contain "nonfattening" fats and oils or synthetic fat additives that pass through the digestive tract unabsorbed. Such fats or oils prevent the absorption of a variety of fat-soluble nutrients. Evidence of indigestible fat in the diet can often be seen in the embarrassing telltale brown stains from the oil that seeps into underclothing.

This is one more good reason your diet should be made up of fresh, natural foods.

Watch Out for Cortisone!

If you have osteoporosis and also suffer from asthma, arthritis, or some other condition that's treated with cortisone, be sure to inform the treating physician that you have osteoporosis. It's well known that excessive or prolonged use of cortisone or corticosteroids can lead to the development of osteoporosis. When osteoporosis is already present, use of cortisone will hasten collapse of already weakened vertebrae.

How Marion P. Halted the Progress of Osteoporosis Caused by Cortisone

Seventy-year-old Marion P. began to complain about upper back pain several weeks after recovering from a bad case of shingles, a virus that also causes chicken pox. "You have post-herpetic neuralgia [residual pain caused by viral infection of a nerve root]," her physician told her, and he prescribed cortisone. When she visited my office a few months later, it was apparent from the slump in her spine, the location of her pain, and the X-ray findings that her worsening back pain was the result of osteoporosis. Three of her thoracic vertebrae, in the middle of her upper back, had already partially collapsed.

When I informed Marion's physician about her osteoporosis, he took her off cortisone (which would further soften her bones) and put her on calcium, vitamin D, and estrogen. I recommended special exercises. The progress of the disease was halted, and there was no further collapse of vertebrae.

Once a vertebra has collapsed from osteoporosis, it remains collapsed, even if the progress of the disease stops. So the hump in Marion's back was permanent. It was fortunate for her, however, that the disease was detected and treated before her entire spine telescoped into a crippling deformity.

Take a look in the mirror and see if you think you are developing a hump on your back. Has your height decreased an inch or two over the past few years? Of course, as you grow older, your height will gradually decrease from dehydration and degeneration of intervertebral discs. But when a sudden decrease in height is associated with development of a humpback, chances are that osteoporosis is involved, especially if your back hurts. Periodontal disease, though most often the result of gum infection, is also sometimes an early sign of osteoporosis.

If you are over sixty years of age and you suspect that you might have osteoporosis, ask your doctor to order an X-ray examination of your thoracic spine. There are also special instruments that can measure the density of bone.

Strengthen Your Back Bones and Your Back Muscles with Special Exercises

Although a back support is often prescribed as a temporary measure in the treatment of vertebral fractures, herniated discs, and low-back sprains, it's often a mistake to use a back support in the treatment of osteoporosis—except in severe cases. Remember that bones are *strengthened* by movement and *weakened* by rest. Some older people develop osteoporosis simply because they are inactive. Wearing a back support or brace makes their muscles even more inactive, further reducing stimulating stress on the vertebrae. Almost any kind of exercise, even raking the yard, will help strengthen bones. A back support restricts movement and limits the weight-bearing function and may weaken vertebrae by depriving them of the stimulation they need to retain and absorb calcium.

Whether you have osteoporosis or not, you should exercise regularly to strengthen your muscles and stimulate your bones. Regular pulling and tugging of muscles on your bones will force them to retain greater amounts of calcium in order to stay strong enough to withstand daily stress.

Four Simple Back Exercises

Exercises involving forced flexion, or bending over, of the spine, such as toe touching and sit-ups, should be avoided when osteoporosis has resulted in collapse of a vertebra. It's important, however, to strengthen muscles on the front as well as the back of the spine for even support.

If you are recovering from a back injury, you should be as active as possible after two to four days of rest, but you may have to wait a few weeks before you begin doing exercises to strengthen your trunk muscles.

I do not generally recommend stretching exercises as a treatment for back pain. Simple muscle contraction or resistive exercise (use of muscles against resistance) through a normal and full range of movement for muscle strengthening is best for protecting the spine.

Here are a few special exercises you can do safely to straighten your spine while you strengthen your muscles. (See Chapter 7 for a personalized back-building program.)

1. **Straight-Arm Pullover:** This exercise will help prevent or counteract the slump that tends to develop in the upper back. Lie on your back with a small throw cushion under your back between your shoulder blades. Hold a light weight (about 5 pounds) in each hand at arm's length, starting over your chest. Bring the weights back over your head and lower them to the floor while inhaling deeply. Return to starting position and repeat ten to twelve times. Keep your arms straight throughout the exercise.

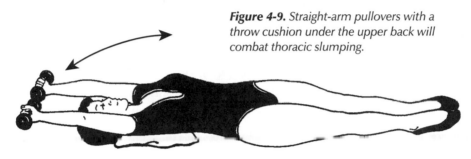

Figure 4-9. Straight-arm pullovers with a throw cushion under the upper back will combat thoracic slumping.

2. **Supine Bent-Knee Leg Lift:** It's important to strengthen your hip-flexor (psoas) and abdominal (rectus abdominis) muscles without placing pressure on vertebrae that have been weakened by osteoporosis.

    Lie on your back with your arms at your sides, your knees bent, and feet flat on the floor. Lift your legs up toward your chest while holding your knees in a bent position. Exhale while lifting your legs. Repeat several times.

3. **Prone One-Leg Lift:** You can use this exercise to tone and strengthen low-back and gluteal (buttock) muscles without placing a strain on your spine.

    Lie face down and raise one straight leg up as high as you can several times. Exercise both legs equally.

4. **Prone Upper Body Arch-Up:** A correctly performed hyperextension exercise will relieve compression on your vertebrae and strengthen important muscles up and down your back.

Lie face down with your feet anchored under a heavy sofa. Without using your arms, lift your upper body from the floor within a comfortable range of movement. Repeat this eight to ten times.

Can Stress Cause Backache?

It's well-known among doctors that anxiety or stress can trigger a backache. It's not clearly understood why or how, but there is evidence to indicate that muscles tightened by stress can result in all kinds of aches and pains. If there also happens to be some arthritis, disc degeneration, or other structural problem in the spine, the muscle tightness can lead to irritation of joints.

Exercise, a hot bath, massage, or a little spinal stretching might relieve symptoms caused by a "nervous backache." Be sure to read Chapter 5 for instructions on how to loosen your spine at home and try the exercises described in Chapter 7.

Any kind of exercise, such as riding a bicycle or swimming, is a great tension reliever. Exercise will also burn off the excess adrenalin produced by emotional stress. Unburned adrenalin, like the cortisone prescribed by a doctor, can draw calcium from your bones. So the next time a stressful situation gets your adrenalin flowing, go out and take a little exercise. Your back muscles will relax as the stress eases, and you'll feel relaxed and rejuvenated.

How Diana K. Relieved Her Tension-type Bachache with Exercise

Diana K. suffered from a tension-type backache that persisted unrelieved until she learned how to relax her mind and her muscles with recreational-type exercise. "All the expensive medical tests and medications I've had over the years did no good at all," she recalled. "Since I've been taking regular exercise, my backache has disappeared—and it's not costing me a cent!"

As Diana learned from experience, unrelieved tension in back muscles can lead to inflammation of muscle fibers (myositis, myofascitis, fibromyositis), which can cause painful spasm. Fibromyalgia is currently a popular diagnosis for generalized muscle pain and could have a systemic, or internal, origin. Rest, exercise, moist heat, massage, cold packs, or any of the backache remedies described in this book may provide relief. *Prevention* is the best treatment. So be sure to do all you can to stay fit, flexible, relaxed, and healthy.

SPECIAL TREATMENTS FOR BACK PAIN

Here are some noninvasive treatment methods that your doctor might be able to use to relieve the symptoms of back pain.

■ **Manipulation** of the spine (manual movement of vertebrae) can be helpful in relieving acute back pain during the first month of symptoms. It can sometimes result in dramatic relief of pain when mobility is restored in spinal joints that are locked or stiffened by adhesions or degenerative changes. A chiropractor, osteopath, physiatrist, or physical therapist can generally provide appropriate manipulation as well as treatment using such modalities as ultrasound, electrical stimulation, or diathermy.

■ **Ultrasound** uses high-frequency sound waves to generate heat and to hasten absorption of waste products deep within injured tissues. It is often used for a couple of weeks to relieve symptoms, followed by use of hot and cold packs at home as needed. Family physicians can sometimes provide treatment with ultrasound.

■ **Electrical stimulation,** in which a mild electrical current is applied by placing electrodes over the painful area, is often used to relieve pain by modifying pain perception. It is also used to stimulate healing of fractures and to cause muscle contraction that will flush out injured muscle fibers. When used as a treatment for injury, it must be applied by a health-care provider such as a physical therapist.

■ **Diathermy** uses high-frequency radio shortwaves or microwaves to generate heat in deep tissues for pain relief or to speed healing. Because of the danger of burns, this is a closely supervised treatment commonly used by physical therapists.

■ **Special exercises** may be needed to restore structural integrity after a back injury and to prevent recurring episodes of back pain. If you do not recover fully after thirty to ninety days of simple exercise, see a doctor who specializes in back care and have him prescribe exercises that are tailored to meet your needs. Back pain that lasts longer than three months is considered to be chronic and may require special stretching and strengthening exercises to eliminate residual weakness, tightness, and stiffness in muscles and joints.

Manipulation Versus Medication

According to the U.S. Department of Health and Human Services' most recent edition of *Guidelines to Acute Low Back Problems in Adults* (1994), spinal manipulation can be effective in relieving nonspecific acute lower back symptoms not accompanied by radiculopathy (damaging nerve pain) when used during the first month of symptoms. "Relief of discomfort can be accomplished most safely with nonprescription medication and/or spinal manipulation," the guidelines report.

A good chiropractor or osteopath who performs spinal manipulation by hand may be able to help you avoid taking prescription medication if your back pain is not incapacitating or accompanied by severe sciatica. (Chiropractors do 94 percent of all the spinal manipulation performed in the United States.[3]) Manipulation should not be continued for longer than one month, however, if symptoms are not relieved. In rare cases, a weakened lumbar disc might herniate into the spinal canal when manipulation is too forceful, causing loss of bladder or bowel control. If this happens, it should immediately be brought to the attention of a neurosurgeon.

Chronic back pain, usually defined as lasting longer than three months, can often be relieved by spinal manipulation as needed; that is, when symptoms indicate a need for such treatment.

When you have difficulty sleeping at night, or when you can hardly get out of bed to go to the bathroom because of acute back pain, a little over-the-counter medication can often relieve your misery. Acute sciatica, or leg pain caused by impingement of a spinal nerve, might require prescription medication for relief of pain. Don't get into the habit of taking pain medication or anti-inflammatory drugs for every little ache or pain, however.

Government guidelines report that extended use of high-dose opioids (prescription pain pills) and prolonged bed rest in the treatment of back pain can prolong symptoms and increase debilitation. Acetaminophen, such as Tylenol, is believed to have fewer side effects and is recommended for pain relief, with bed rest limited to four days.

Note: Prolonged use of acetaminophen can lead to liver damage.

Nonsteroidal anti-inflammatory drugs, such as aspirin or ibuprofen, can relieve pain as well as reduce inflammation. Remember, however, that all anti-inflammatory drugs tend to irritate the stomach and can cause gastrointestinal bleeding. Obviously, you should take medication only when necessary and for only as long as necessary. I personally prefer aspirin for its combined pain relief and anti-inflammatory effects (and its tendency to prevent heart attacks caused by blood clots), but only occasionally and only for a few days at a time. Discontinue the use of aspirin if you have any kind of surgery scheduled, especially back surgery.

When you have severe pain or throbbing inflammation and over-the-counter drugs do not seem to help, your doctor might prescribe a more potent painkiller (such as an opioid analgesic) or an anti-inflammatory drug (such as a corticosteroid) along with a cold pack. Government guidelines report, however, that opioids appear to be no more effective than acetaminophen or aspirin in relieving lower back pain and may be addictive.

Muscle relaxants have not been shown to be more effective than aspirin and other nonsteroidal anti-inflammatory drugs. Remember that muscle spasm is a reflex protective mechanism and probably should not be suppressed through the use of medication. Muscle relaxants are therefore not recommended.

Note: Some prescription muscle relaxants have been known to result in urinary retention, which might be mistaken for cauda equina, a syndrome caused by massive lumbar disc herniation into the spinal canal. Be sure to let your doctor know if you are taking a muscle relaxant and you have urinary control or retention problems.

Your body produces its own painkilling endorphins, which can be stimulated by manipulation, massage, hot packs, or cold packs. Use of spinal manipulation and self-help remedies is a form of *active* treatment that will speed recovery much more rapidly than passive bed rest and pain medication.

In the next chapter, I'll describe a few vertebrae-loosening techniques that you can use at home to relieve stiffness and binding in your spine.

SUMMARY

1. Most of the time, low-back pain is the result of simple strain, but disc herniations and other serious back problems occur most often in the lower spine.

2. Resting on a firm mattress with your knees bent and using occasional moist heat applications will often relieve Type M back pain.

3. A wrap-around, Velcro-fastening lumbar support may be helpful in supporting or protecting a painful or unstable spine.

4. Pain and numbness radiating down one leg, especially when preceded or accompanied by back pain, might be an indication of disc herniation.

5. Weakness or loss of sensation in the foot, ankle, leg, or thigh, or the shrinking of leg muscles, should be brought to the attention of a neurologist.

6. Stretching your back at home, with or without apparatus, will often relieve painful pressure on joints, discs, and nerves.

7. Curvatures and structural abnormalities in the spine can cause chronic or recurring back pain, which must be differentiated from other more serious problems, such as osteoporosis.

8. You should always suspect osteoporosis if you are an elderly woman with chronic backache, especially if you have a hump in your upper back.

9. Unrelieved stress and tension can cause backache and muscle spasm by tightening and inflaming back muscles.

10. People suffering from increasingly severe or unrelieved backache should not assume their problem is caused by arthritis or some other previously diagnosed Type M back problem. Always get an updated diagnosis.

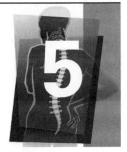

How You Can Loosen and Align Your Spinal Joints Safely and Effectively

We all want to be youthful and flexible. We interpret stiffness as a sign of old age and poor physical conditioning. There is plenty you can do at home to improve and maintain flexibility, and you will improve your health in the process.

While most of this chapter is focused on the spine, it also describes special exercises designed to take the tightness out of the muscles and tendons that have an influence on movement and support of the spine. Tight hamstrings, for example, may limit forward bending, even if the spine itself is flexible. Tight hip flexors can contribute to swayback, causing lower back pain as well as poor posture, and so on.

Many of the exercises designed to stretch out tightness and loosen vertebrae are invigorating and will provide you with a sense of well-being. A back massage technique designed to relieve tension and relax muscles also provides pure pleasure. When there is discomfort associated with stiffness in spinal joints, special back-loosening techniques will provide welcome relief. All of this can be done safely and effectively at home. If you need a good chiropractor to loosen a kinked neck or back, I'll even tell you how to find one.

The techniques described in this chapter will provide pleasure as well as improve your physical condition. And you'll want to make everything you learn in this chapter a permanent part of a self-help program designed to ease tension and backache at the end of a long day.

The Mystery of Cracking Joints

Most of us instinctively try to crack our back when we have a "catch" in our spine. We bend, move, and stretch our vertebrae until we feel that welcome click that seems to release the binding and tightness that is causing us discomfort.

What is that mysterious crack? It's probably not what you think it is; it's certainly not always a vertebra out of place (see Chapter 14). If you feel a little cracking or clicking in your spine while doing some of the stretching and loosening exercises described in this chapter, that doesn't necessarily mean that your vertebrae are slipping into or out of place.

Actually, your vertebrae are securely fastened to each other by interlocking joints, strong ligaments, and tough intervertebral disc fibers. A normal joint cannot easily slip out of place unless there has been disease or injury in joints, discs, or ligaments. So don't worry about your vertebrae slipping around when you exercise. You can safely relieve or avoid stiffness or discomfort by doing the spinal-loosening exercises described in this chapter. Properly performed exercise will, in fact, keep your vertebrae better aligned by maintaining normal mobility.

When there is a binding or locking in a spinal joint, there might be a click or a cracking sound when the joint suddenly becomes released or loosened. You can also make a perfectly normal and freely moving joint crack, just as when you crack your knuckles.

Basically, spinal joint surfaces move over each other like two wet glass slides. While the joints slide over each other quite easily, they do not easily separate because of the attraction between the two wet, smooth surfaces. When these joints are forced to separate by manipulation or stretching, the fluid attraction between the joint surfaces is broken, causing a cracking sound. Since the separation produces a vacuum in the joint, gases are released to fill the space, just as carbon dioxide is released when you pop a champagne cork. The capsule surrounding the joint might also snap in a little. Once a joint cracks, it might be a few minutes or hours before it will crack again—after the gas has been absorbed and the joint surfaces settle back together.

Of course, this breaking apart of joint surfaces loosens tight joints by tearing apart adhesions and improving lubrication. It might also relieve irritation or pinching of joint cartilage or a joint capsule. In either case, it's clear that a joint is not always out of place just because it cracks.

Don't Get Hooked on Joint Popping

Some joints crack more readily than others, depending upon the angle of joint surfaces, the viscosity of joint fluids, the curve of the spine, the person's age, the amount of muscle tightness and nervous tension, and other factors. Inability to relax, for example, makes it difficult to crack joints in some portions of the spine, even though the joints can be made to slide over each other with mobilization techniques.

Joint cracking heard during spinal manipulation is normally not significant or harmful. Excessive cracking, however, can irritate a joint, and excessive use of spinal manipulation to crack your vertebrae can lead to instability in a spinal joint. When cracking occurs during general loosening procedures done at home to relieve stiffness, that's okay. But you should not seek or undergo professional spinal manipulation unless you have back trouble, nor should you undergo regular spinal manipulation just because your back cracks.

Spinal manipulators who take advantage of the trick of cracking normal joints will often pick out spinal joints that pop easily and then repeatedly manipulate the joints, letting the patient believe that the cracking is evidence that the joints are constantly slipping out of place. Some of these practitioners may also repeatedly X-ray these joints, supposedly measuring the amount of correction resulting from manipulation. This is a useless and dangerous practice. Except in cases where muscle spasm has pulled the spine to one side or a disc has herniated, no change can be seen in X rays following a manipulation, even after months of cracking the vertebrae.

Occasionally, but not very often, an abnormal or unstable spinal joint will slip too far and lock or bind in an abnormal position, causing pain that locks the spine and restricts movement, and this can be seen on X-ray film. When this happens, the joint can usually be released with one manipulation, restoring normal, pain-free movement. It would be pointless to continue with spinal manipulation or to X-ray the spine again.

Spinal Care Without Fear

Spinal X rays can be harmful to the body and should never be taken without good reason—usually only if there are signs of disease or injury or if symptoms persist for longer than four weeks. According to the latest U.S. guidelines published by the Agency for Healthcare Research and Quality, in Rockville, MD, "X rays are not recommended for routine evaluation of patients with acute low back problems within the first month of symptoms unless a red flag is noted on clinical examination." Thermography, a procedure that measures and compares temperature differences on both sides of the body, which is commonly offered free by some chiropractors to locate "pinched nerves" prior to X-ray examination, "...is not recommended for assessing patients with acute low back problems.... The one study meeting review criteria found that thermography did not accurately predict either the presence or absence of lumbar nerve root compression found at surgery.... Based on the available research evidence, thermography does not appear effective for diagnosing low back problems." So don't let anyone convince you that you need extensive X-ray examination based on thermography findings. And don't be led to believe that you need regular professional manipulation just because your back cracks.

Once it has been established that recurring back pain is caused by a degenerated disc, arthritic stiffness, spinal curvature, or joint abnormality that is contributing to binding or fixation of a vertebral joint, manipulation can be repeated as needed without repeated X-ray examination.

Some of the exercises described in this chapter are designed to loosen and align your spinal joints. That doesn't mean, however, that you should be concerned or obsessed with cracking your vertebrae. An occasional back-popping manipulation, when properly performed, feels great, especially when done by a competent chiropractor, and it may improve flexibility in your spine. When the spine is tight and stiff, spinal manipulation provides relaxing relief. But you should be on guard to avoid becoming a life-long patient of a spinal manipulator who cracks normal joints to "prevent disease" by removing imaginary nerve interference or an elusive "pinched nerve." There is no credible evidence that a vertebra out of alignment can cause disease or that manipulation of the spine can cure or prevent disease.

Prevention Is Your Responsibility!

If you exercise regularly, keep yourself flexible, and maintain good posture, you're less likely to have back trouble and less likely to need spinal manipulation. Prevention is something *you* must do, not your doctor. It's up to you to keep your back strong and your spine flexible in order to *prevent* back trouble.

When mechanical-type back trouble does occur, spinal manipulation provided by a chiropractor can be an effective treatment. Since a large number of chiropractors, in keeping with the basic tenets of chiropractic, use spinal manipulation as a method of "restoring and maintaining health," requiring prolonged and often unnecessary treatment (see Chapter 14), it's necessary to look for a chiropractor who has a properly limited practice (see the first bullet in the sidebar below for a description of what I mean by this).

FINDING A GOOD CHIROPRACTOR

A good chiropractor who uses spinal manipulation appropriately can do much to help you with neck and back pain and related ailments, such as tension headache and muscle and joint tightness. But you must choose carefully. A good chiropractor

- has a practice that is limited to the treatment of neuromusculoskeletal problems of mechanical origin;
- uses physical therapy modalities as well as spinal manipulation;
- performs spinal manipulation manually and does not use an instrument to adjust "subluxated (misaligned) vertebrae";
- does not routinely X-ray new patients and uses X ray only when necessary;
- provides a diagnosis rather than a "spinal analysis";
- does not require payment in advance for a series of treatments;
- treats patients as needed and discharges them when they are symptom-free;
- does not offer spinal manipulation as a method of restoring and maintaining health and does not use "spinal adjustments" as a preventive measure;
- does not advertise free exams to attract new patients;
- will work with your family physician or a medical specialist, exchanging office notes when necessary; or
- does not treat infants or toddlers or children under the age of twelve unless referred by a pediatrician or an orthopedist.

Your family physician, an orthopedist, or a neurologist can sometimes help you locate a good chiropractor.

I'll tell you how to loosen your spinal joints in this chapter, but first let's do something to relieve the tightness in the muscles supporting your spine.

Stretching Ankle, Thigh, Hip, and Back Muscles

The muscles supporting your spine function like the guy wires that hold up a television antenna (before cable TV, that is). The tension of muscles on the front, back, and each side of the spine, when equal, holds the spine erect and balanced. When one set of muscles is weak, uneven muscle tension tends to pull the spine off balance, causing aches and pains in muscles and joints.

Muscles that are too short will result in spinal tilting or tugging that overworks the opposing set of muscles. Persons who do not exercise regularly usually have weak abdominal muscles and tight hip flexors. These weak or shortened muscles do not adequately balance the strength of low-back muscles, which are kept fairly strong from everyday use.

You'll learn more about muscle imbalance when you read the material on posture in Chapter 9. In this chapter, we'll be concerned primarily with stretching tight leg and back muscles and loosening a stiff spine.

How Cheryl B.'s Short Ankle Tendons Caused Back and Leg Ache

Cheryl B. had been experiencing backache and leg ache for several months when she first visited my office. "At the end of the day," she complained, "my back and legs ache so badly that I can hardly finish eight hours on the job. I've never had such a backache before."

Taking Cheryl's history, I learned that she had previously worked as a sales clerk in a dress shop. It wasn't until she switched to her present job in a fast-food restaurant that she began to experience backache and leg ache. When her physical examination revealed that she had unusually tight hamstrings and short ankle tendons, I asked her about the type of shoes she had been wearing. "I wore high-heeled shoes when I worked in the dress shop," she answered, "but I switched to low heels when I started working in the restaurant."

After negative X rays and a little detective work, it became apparent that Cheryl's backache was caused by tight leg muscles that were pulling on her lower back. Years of wearing high-heeled shoes had contributed to shortening of ankle tendons and hamstrings. Sudden lowering of her heels by switching to low-heeled shoes was creating muscle tension that was pulling from her heels to her back. In an unconscious effort to ease the pull on her ankle tendons, she was developing a slew-footed stance, with her feet pointing outward on each side instead of straight ahead. This was causing an inward rolling of her ankles and knees, which was tilting her pelvis to produce a sway back, further increasing the pull on tight hamstrings.

These sudden changes in body mechanics were resulting in inflammation and spasm of low-back muscles, as well as jamming of lower lumbar facets (joints).

I gave Cheryl some stretching exercises and advised her to switch to shoes with higher heels.

"Simply changing shoes has greatly relieved my backache," Cheryl reported. "But I intend to do the stretching exercises to get the tightness out of my legs."

The lesson in Cheryl's story is that even though wearing high-heeled shoes may be bad for your back, you cannot suddenly switch from high heels to low heels if you have been wearing high-heeled shoes for a number of years. The change should be made gradually, with special stretching exercises to lengthen shortened muscles and tendons on the back of the ankles and calves.

Two Simple Tests for Short Hamstrings and Ankle Tendons

Straight-leg raise test: Lie flat on your back and raise one leg straight up as high as you can. If you cannot raise each leg higher than 45 degrees because of pulling behind your knees, chances are your hamstrings are too tight. Restriction in both legs points to tight hamstrings, while restriction in one leg might be an indication of a sciatic nerve problem.

The ankle-flexion test: Sit upright on the floor with your legs locked straight out in front of you. If you cannot flex the top of both feet past a right angle toward your shins, your ankle tendons may be too short. If your hamstrings are also tight, you'll find it difficult to straighten your legs out in front while sitting upright on the floor to test your ankle tendons. If so, just lean backward until you can lock your legs out straight then flex the top of your foot toward your shin.

Three Ways to Stretch Tight Ankle Tendons

The wall stretch: Stand at arm's length from a wall, facing the wall. Place both hands on the wall. Lean toward the wall by bending your elbows while keeping your body straight and both feet flat on the floor. You should be able to feel your ankle tendons stretching. Be sure to keep your toes pointed straight ahead and your heels on the floor.

The heel drop: Stand with the balls of both feet on a low step or a thick board and lower your heels to the floor. Rise up on your toes and again lower your heels to the floor. Repeat several times, gradually increasing the number of repetitions over a period of several weeks.

The donkey exercise: For an even greater stretch on ankle tendons, bend over from a standing position and brace both hands on a chair seat. Lower your heels from a thick board that's supporting the balls of both feet. Begin with only a few repetitions and gradually increase the number as you become accustomed to the stretch.

How to Stretch Tight Hamstrings

You can stretch tight hamstrings simply by lying on your back and raising one straight leg as high as you can. You may also sit on the floor and lean forward while your legs are locked straight out. You can force some additional stretch by grasping your legs with your hands and pulling with your arms while leaning forward.

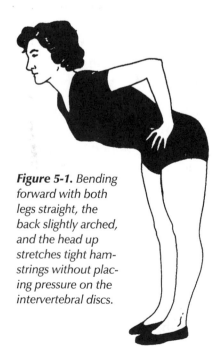

Figure 5-1. Bending forward with both legs straight, the back slightly arched, and the head up stretches tight hamstrings without placing pressure on the intervertebral discs.

The good morning exercise: Probably the best way to stretch tight hamstrings without placing compression on spinal discs is to place both hands on your hips and bend forward with your head up and a slight arch in your lower back. Keep your spine straight and flat while bending so that movement takes place only in the hip joints. Bend forward until you feel your hamstrings stretch.

If you have a low-back problem or a herniated disc, you should not do straight-leg toe-touching exercises in a standing position. If you do toe-touching exercises of any kind, they should not be done so rapidly that the momentum created forces excessive forward bending of the spine, placing excessive compression on spinal discs. Bending the knees during toe touching will reduce compression on spinal discs.

Tight Thigh Bands Can Cause Backache

People who sit all day and do not exercise will often develop a tightness in the layers of fascia that cover the muscles on the outside of the thighs. This tightness in iliotibial "thigh bands" is a common but little recognized cause of backache.

A Test for Tight Thigh Bands

Lie on your side and pull the knee on the bottom side up toward your abdomen. Bend the knee of the upper leg (placing the foot of that leg behind you) and move the leg backward. Relax and let the upper leg sag. If the knee of the upper leg will not drop low enough to touch the floor, your thigh bands may be too tight.

How to Stretch Tight Thigh Bands

Stand at arm's length from a wall, with the wall to your side. Reach out and place your hand against the wall. Bend the elbow of the supporting arm and lean toward the wall. Bend your trunk toward the wall so that you stretch the outside of the thigh that's next to the wall. Stretch both sides several times. Try to keep your beltline horizontal to the floor for more effective stretching.

Stretching Hip Flexors to Prevent Backache

The iliopsoas muscles, also called hip flexors (the "filet mignon" muscles), are responsible for flexing the hips, that is, lifting the thighs. Attached between the lumbar vertebrae and the top of the femur or thigh bones, these muscles are sometimes so short that they literally pull the lumbar spine into a sway-backed posture during standing.

Unfortunately, the role of the hip flexors in the development of backache is often overlooked. Many of the exercises prescribed in the treatment of backache are flexion-type exercises that contribute even more to shortening of the hip flexors. Sit-ups, for example, require contraction of hip flexors. Any exercise in which the trunk is moved forward by muscle contraction that bends the hips involves the hip flexors. Simply sitting for long periods of time may contribute to shortening of hip flexors.

When you have an acutely painful low-back problem, the pain you feel in your lower back when you attempt to do a sit-up or lift your thighs is usually caused by the pull of hip flexors on the lower lumbar vertebrae. You'll learn from experience to avoid the use of your hip flexors when back pain is acute.

Bend Your Knees During Sit-ups!

Even when you aren't having back pain, you can protect your back by avoiding excessive leverage or pull on your hip flexors. This is why sit-ups and leg raises should be done with the knees *bent*. If bent-knee sit-ups cause back pain as well, you should avoid use of your hip flexors by doing trunk curls instead of sit-ups.

In a trunk curl, you simply curl your head and shoulders up from the floor, contracting only your abdominal muscles. Any attempt to sit up by lifting your lower back off the floor would require contraction of your hip flexors.

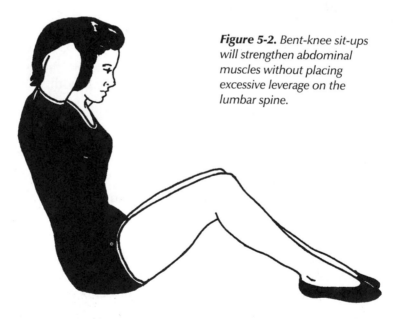

Figure 5-2. Bent-knee sit-ups will strengthen abdominal muscles without placing excessive leverage on the lumbar spine.

How to Stretch Hip Flexors by Extending Your Thighs

Since most of us sit too much, shortened hip flexors are common. It's therefore a good idea to stretch your hip flexors with regular exercise, especially if you do sit-ups.

Any exercise in which you must extend or move one thigh back while flexing or moving one thigh forward, as in doing a split, will stretch hip flexors on the side of the thigh moving back. You must be careful, however, not to strain your hips with excessive stretching or splitting.

The kneeling lunge: Simple kneeling lunges might be the simplest and easiest way to stretch hip flexors without a strain on your lumbar spine. Begin in a kneeling position with your weight supported on the knee of one leg and on the foot of the other leg out in front. With your knee and your foot securely anchored, shift your body weight forward by bending the uppermost knee. Keep your upper body as vertical as possible in order to increase the stretch on hip flexors on the side of the extending thigh. Stretch both sides equally by switching leg positions.

Note: Pain caused by nerve root impingement in the upper portion of the lumbar spine, causing radiation down one of the femoral nerves on the *front* of the thigh, may be aggravated by hip and thigh extension in a kneeling lunge. Be sure to see a doctor if you have persistent aching, numbness, or tingling that seems to radiate down the front of one of your thighs.

Stretching Tight Back Muscles

You can stretch tight muscles up and down your back simply by lying on your side and rolling up into a ball, pulling your knees up toward your head.

Side Bending for Side Muscles

Although the muscles on each side of your trunk rarely get tight enough to cause backache, it wouldn't hurt to do a little side bending for all-around flexibility.

Stand erect with your hands on your hips and bend from side to side. Do this exercise slowly to avoid excessive and possibly damaging momentum.

Stretching Rib Cage Muscles

The rib cage and its supporting muscles offer important support for the thoracic spine. It's important to lift and stretch the rib cage with special exercises to reduce the tendency of the thoracic spine to slump. (The isotonic straight-arm pullover described in Chapter 4, used in the prevention of dowager's hump, is a good stretching exercise that extends the thoracic spine.)

You may be able to stretch your rib cage effectively by doing an isometric bent-arm sofa lift. Lie on your back, reach back over your head with both arms, and hook both hands under the bottom of a heavy sofa or a cedar chest. Inhale deeply while exerting pressure with your arms, as if trying to lift the sofa. Keep your abdominal muscles relaxed and your elbows bent while lifting your rib cage as high as you can. You should be able to feel your chest muscles lift your rib cage to accommodate your expanding lungs.

Remember that the exercises described in this chapter are designed to *stretch* tight muscles. You'll learn in Chapter 7 how to *strengthen* the muscles that support your spine. Select the exercises you think you need most.

How to Loosen Your Vertebrae

Unlike exercises designed to stretch or strengthen muscles, vertebrae-loosening exercises require very little muscle contraction. In fact, vertebral joints actually loosen best when they are forced to move in postures in which the muscles are *totally relaxed*. This is why spinal manipulators insist on complete relaxation by the patient during manipulation.

Any kind of exercise that requires movement of the spinal joints will keep the spine in its natural alignment. But when portions of the spine have been stiffened by arthritis, or when spinal curvatures and other structural abnormalities restrict normal movement in some of the joints of the spine, special loosening exercises will help unlock joints and relieve stiffness.

Don't do any exercise that causes pain. Spinal-loosening exercises should feel good. Any cracking that occurs during a loosening should be painless. If you have arthritis, osteoporosis, or some other painful spinal problem, or if you have suffered a painful back injury, don't do any of the exercises in this chapter without your doctor's permission.

Vertebrae-loosening exercises are designed primarily to relieve stiffness and to maintain the mobility you need to stay flexible and healthy and not to relieve acute pain.

Warm Up and Loosen Up with the Camel-Horse Exercise

The easiest way to loosen your spine is to do the camel-horse exercise.

Get down on your hands and knees. Arch your back up (like a camel) while lowering your head. Then arch your back down (like a sway-backed horse) while lifting your head. Arch up and down several times—until you feel warm and loose.

This exercise will move all of your spinal joints a little, and it will relieve pressure on your intervertebral discs.

Figure 5-3. *Arching your back up and down for several repetitions while on your hands and knees will warm up muscles and loosen vertebrae.*

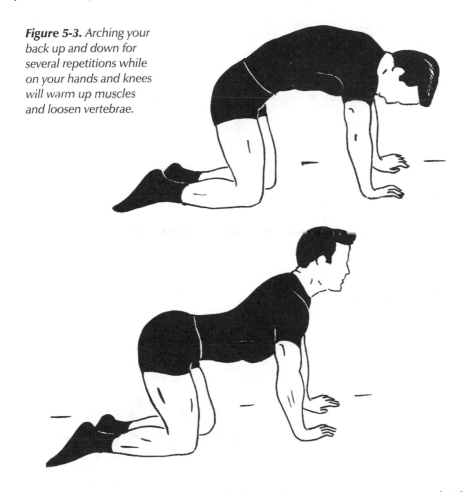

The soft center, or nucleus, of a disc is about 90 percent water at birth. After the age of twenty-five or thirty, the discs begin to dry out, making them thinner and stiffer. When you do the camel-horse exercise, the up and down tilting of your vertebrae moves fluid inside the discs without any weight-bearing compression on your spine. This movement of fluid and the stretching of disc fibers tends to keep the discs strong and elastic, improving flexibility in your spine.

When your spine is stiff from lying in bed or from sitting or standing too long, take a few minutes and do the camel-horse exercise before resorting to the use of aspirin or some other medication. Chances are that the exercise will relieve your nagging aches and pains and you won't need to take medication.

If this exercise doesn't do the job, you can try one that's more specific for your upper back or your lower back, depending on where your pain is located.

The Upper-Back Carpet Roll Adjustment

Because of the pull of gravity and the natural tendency of the spine to slump, fatigue sometimes results in uncomfortable binding of rib joints and vertebral joints in the thoracic spine. Most of us will automatically try to relieve this binding by moving our shoulders back in an effort to pop our vertebrae. When you must sit for a long time in a straight-backed chair, chances are you'll occasionally lean backward to relieve fatigue by forcefully extending your spine.

The more slumping there is in your spine, the greater the tendency for your spine to ache from postural fatigue. You might be able to relieve this aching by "adjusting" your spine with a carpet roll. Don't do this exercise, however, if you have acute back pain or if you have osteoporosis.

Figure 5-4. Lying over a roll of carpet padding in this carpet roll exercise will loosen and extend the thoracic spine.

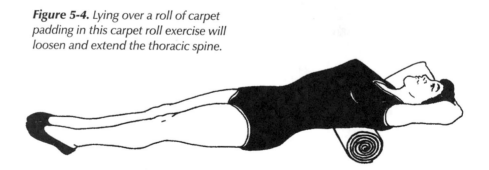

Carpet padding makes a good soft roll. You can also use a rolled up blanket or some other soft material.

Make a roll that's four or five inches in diameter and about two feet long. Lay the roll on a carpeted floor and then lie over the roll so that it supports your upper back across your shoulder blades. Relax for several seconds and let the weight of your body and the pressure of the roll extend or flatten your spine. Placing your hands behind your head will increase extension of your spine.

How Peter T. and Ron B. Relieved Back and Chest Pain with a Carpet Roll Adjustment

Peter T. spent several hours a day working as a draftsman for a busy architect. "I sit slumped over a drawing board all day," Peter explained, "so my upper back gets real tired and stiff. I made a roll out of carpet padding that I keep in my office. When my back starts hurting, I lie down on the roll for a few minutes to relieve my pain and then I go back to work. I don't believe I could get by without my carpet roll."

Ron B. had been having chest pain for several weeks. Examinations by cardiologists and internists had ruled out a heart or lung problem, but the pain persisted. Ron discovered accidentally that using a carpet roll would relieve his chest pain.

"When I used a carpet roll to ease my backache," Ron recalled, "my back popped and my chest pain disappeared! I still feel the pain occasionally, but it always goes away when I use the carpet roll."

Ron's chest pain was caused by nerve root irritation in an arthritic spine. When he loosened his upper spine with the carpet roll treatment, the nerve pinching was relieved, thus relieving the chest pain that was being referred into his rib cage.

The Supine Low-Back Twist

The joints of the lower spine are shaped primarily to move back and forth, as in bending forward or backward. But when the joints of the lower spine are stiff, fixed, or locked, a rotating movement seems to be most effective in breaking them loose.

The most common manipulation used on the lower spine by professionals is a form of rotation combined with a stretch. It is this type of manipulation that most often produces a crack in the lower back. Properly performed, such manipulation is safe and effective. When inappropriate or improperly performed, however, it can be a potentially harmful treatment. So don't ever try to crack someone else's back by twisting his or her spine. You can, however, safely loosen your own spine by performing a simple loosening exercise that requires rotation of your lower back.

Caution: Do not do the low-back twist if it causes pain or discomfort. Be especially cautious if you have leg pain.

The low-back twist: Lie flat on your back with your arms spread out or at your sides. Bend your knees and lift your feet off the floor. Hold your legs together in this bent position and lower them first to one side and then to the other side by twisting at your waist. Keep your upper back flat on the floor in order to increase the amount of rotation in your lower spine.

Figure 5-5. Lowering the legs from side to side in a supine low-back twist stretches tight back muscles and loosens lumbar vertebrae.

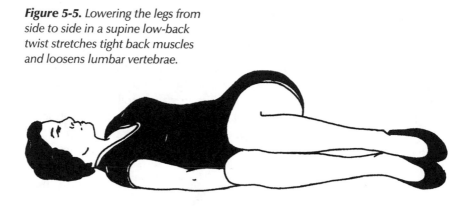

Each time you lower your legs to the floor, relax your muscles for a couple of seconds so that the weight of your legs forces additional rotation of your lower lumbar vertebrae.

How Ann P. Uses the Low-Back Twist to Realign Her Spine

Ann P. is convinced that some of her lumbar vertebrae are slipping out of alignment when she develops a low-back pain after bowling. "My back frequently goes out when I bowl," she observed. "All I have to do to get it back in place is to lie on my back and twist from side to side."

Like many people who suffer from recurring back trouble, Ann has discovered that she can benefit from spinal loosening exercises at home.

How to Give a Professional Sofa Cushion Adjustment

If you have a partner or mate who can work on your back, you might want to try a sofa cushion adjustment when your back is tight and aching. Try the adjustment on your partner before having your partner try it on you.

Place three sofa cushions end to end on the floor and have your partner lie face down on the cushions with his/her chin hanging over the top edge of the first cushion. Both forearms should rest on the floor alongside the cushions.

Straddle your partner in a kneeling position and place your hands palm down in the center of your partner's back so that your thumbs are parallel and about one inch apart. Rotate your wrists inward a little so that all of the pressure is on the thick muscle on the thumb side of your palms.

Press downward and slightly headward until the skin is pulled tight and the spine is pressed down. Ask your partner to take a deep breath and then exhale. Maintain pressure on the spine while your partner is exhaling. Then, at the end of the exhalation, push a couple of inches further with a short, quick thrust.

It's important that your partner not hold her breath during the thrust. If she succeeds in relaxing and does not hold her breath during the thrust, there may be audible clicks when the vertebrae move. The clicks should be followed by a sense of relief from tension.

A single thrust between the shoulder blades might be enough to loosen the thoracic vertebrae. You might, however, want to thrust over all the vertebrae that have ribs attached to them. Begin at the shoulders and work down to the waist. Use only a moderate amount of pressure. Don't try to make the vertebrae crack by using more and more force. Even if the vertebrae don't crack, the use of gentle pressure will loosen the spine. Besides, if you or your partner learn to relax during the manipulation, the vertebrae will loosen without the heavy thrust that is automatically resisted by reflex muscle tension.

How Henry B. Uses a Sofa Cushion Adjustment to Ease Pain and Tightness

Henry B., a bus driver, taught his wife to give him a sofa cushion adjustment. "When I have pain and tightness between my shoulder blades at the end of a long trip," Henry reported, "my wife can always relieve my pain by giving me a sofa cushion adjustment. I've saved a fortune in chiropractors' bills by using this manipulation at home!"

The Standing Lift Spinal Adjustment

This is another home spinal adjustment that requires the assistance of a partner. It is a traction-type manipulation that will stretch and loosen vertebrae from the shoulders down. Coaches and trainers often use this manipulation to "stretch out the kinks" in the backs of injured athletes.

Stand behind the person you want to stretch. Instruct the person to cross his arms and place his hands on top of his shoulders. Place a small throw cushion against the person's back and then press your chest against the cushion. Encircle the person's body with your arms and lock your hands under his elbows. Instruct the person to rest his head on one of your shoulders so that he will be totally relaxed.

Lift the person by leaning backward and lifting with your arms while pushing up against the pillow with your chest. When the person's feet are almost off the floor, simultaneously squeeze him against the pillow and push with your chest while lifting him off the floor with a quick tug.

It's important for the person to relax for the stretching to be effective. Also, the person doing the stretching should be a little taller than the person being stretched for best results. Standing on a thick board might help increase height.

What About Cracking the Neck Vertebrae?

Since the neck is such a delicate structure, you should not attempt to manipulate your own or some else's neck. The neck stretching techniques described in Chapter 3 will be enough to stretch tight neck muscles and relieve pressure on spinal joints.

Simply rotating your head from side to side and bending your neck back and forth will adequately move the joints of the cervical spine. You'll learn in Chapter 7 how to strengthen the muscles of your neck with special exercises that will help restore and maintain normal curves in your cervical spine.

You should avoid exercises that place a strain on your neck, such as wrestler's bridges and head stands. Unfortunately, some popular neck exercises are potentially damaging to the cervical spine. Rolling the head around in a circle, for example, might cause neck problems, especially if there is arthritis or a structural abnormality in the cervical vertebrae. I've seen several patients recently who were suffering from recurring neck pain caused by head rolling.

How Nathalie D. Relieved Her Neck Pain by Changing Exercises

When Nathalie D. visited my office for the third time in three months complaining of neck pain, I questioned her about her activities and learned that head rolling was part of her dance and exercise routine. When she quit doing the head rolling, her neck problem disappeared.

"When the head rolling routine comes up," Nathalie said later, "I just turn my head from side to side while everyone else is rolling their heads around. The soreness and the aching have disappeared, and I haven't had a neck spasm since I quit doing the head rolling."

Do Your Stretching Exercises Alone

Use a little common sense when doing exercises that involve group participation. Don't do any exercise that causes discomfort. Stop doing an exercise that causes pain, especially a stretching exercise. Back injuries often occur when stretching exercises are done in group workouts where the individual is pushed too far and tries to keep up with the pace and the ability of the instructor and the others in the group.

Stretching and loosening exercises are best done alone at your own pace so that everything you do will be comfortable for *you*.

Remember that the momentum generated by doing back-stretching exercises too fast is responsible for many strains and injuries. Stretching exercises should always be done slowly and carefully and should be stopped the minute pain or discomfort occurs.

Back Massage at Home

We all enjoy a full body massage. Many of us seek massage for relaxation as well as for pleasure. When you have an ache or a pain in your back, however, localized massage—not full-body massage—is usually what's needed. Such massage can be done at home if you have a mate or a partner who can do it for you.

Actually, massage is not a complicated procedure. You don't have to do all the fancy petrissage (rolling and squeezing), tapotement (pounding and tapping), friction (finger tip circular motions), or vibration (shaking) techniques used by professionals. The muscle goading (probing of muscles with fingers, knuckles, or an elbow) used by some masseurs and masseuses to work out "trigger points" is often painful and counterproductive and probably should not be used at all. I have seen a number of patients who have complained of muscle pain for days after a painful session of Rolfing, a form of goading that attempts to "realign" muscles by stretching connective tissue. I remember one case in particular in which a patient had a muscle weakness in his left shoulder because a masseuse had applied deep, goading pressure with a knuckle to a trapezius muscle. The repeated goading had damaged a nerve that supplied the patient's deltoid (shoulder) muscle, making it impossible for him to lift his arm overhead. Fortunately, the weakness was temporary, and the patient regained full strength in his shoulder when the goading was discontinued.

The point of all this is that massage should never be painful. Massage should make you feel better, not worse. So don't hesitate to tell your masseur or masseuse to discontinue any painful pressure or probing.

When you need localized massage for a sore or injured muscle or joint, simple kneading or effleurage (superficial or deep stroking of muscles) is all that's needed.

A simple back-kneading technique: Cover the area to be massaged with a light coating of oil or lotion. Place one or both hands over the area to be massaged and stroke or knead toward the heart. To massage spinal (spina erecta) muscles, start at the bottom of the back, or just below the painful area, and place one hand on each side of the spine over the ridge of muscle that travels up the back. Knead in short, overlapping strokes, working toward the head. Massage the painful area, or the full length of the spine, three or four times.

Firm, vigorous massage stimulates the production of endorphins, the body's own painkiller. Massage should be gentle and light, however, when the object is the relaxation of muscles. Remember, all you're trying to accomplish with massage is to stimulate venous blood flow in order to flush out waste products and replenish tissue fluids. Massage can be preceded or followed by application of moist heat. Vibrators and machine massagers are not an adequate substitute for the stroking effects of massage.

SUMMARY

1. An audible crack in a spinal joint does not necessarily mean that the joint has slipped in or out of place.

2. You should avoid spinal manipulation in which the object is to crack a spinal joint for the purpose of treating or preventing organic disease.

3. Short ankle tendons, hamstrings, thigh bands, or hip flexors can cause backache by producing an abnormal pelvic tilt.

4. Spinal joints stiffened by adhesions or locked by fixations can produce backache by interfering with normal movement.

5. You can restore normal movement in your spine by stretching supporting muscles and loosening spinal joints with special exercises that can be done at home.

6. Loosening techniques that are designed to relieve binding or locking in spinal joints must be done in postures that permit total relaxation of muscles.

7. The prevention of back trouble, which includes stretching and loosening of your spine, along with exercises to strengthen supporting muscles, is something that must be done by *you,* not by your chiropractor.

8. Do not do any stretching or loosening exercise that causes pain or discomfort.

9. While it's all right to allow a partner to "adjust" your thoracic and lumbar spine with the manipulative techniques described in this chapter, you should never allow anyone but a professional to crack your neck.

10. Do your loosening and stretching exercises at home rather than in classes, where attempts to keep pace with a group might result in an injury.

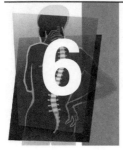

How to Eat to Reduce Body Weight and Relieve Backache

This chapter is based largely upon *Dietary Goals for the United States* and the more recent *Dietary Guidelines for Americans*, which recommend that a large part of your daily calorie intake be provided by fresh, natural carbohydrates (fruits, vegetables, and whole-grain products), the basis for any good, healthful diet—whether you are overweight or not.[4] I recommend, however, that you try to eliminate refined carbohydrates and sugars so that at least *58 percent* of your daily calorie intake comes from natural carbohydrates. I'll tell you how to do that in this chapter.

With six of the ten leading causes of death in the United States linked to diet, there are many good reasons you should follow the healthful *Dietary Guidelines*. One additional important reason is that controlling your body weight will help relieve your backache.

How Wanda T.'s Back Pain Was Being Aggravated by Her Excess Weight

When Wanda first walked into my office, I felt a sense of despair and frustration. Wanda was greatly overweight, and she was obviously suffering from acute back pain. She could barely move. When she sat down in my waiting room, she could not get up by herself.

Whatever the cause of Wanda's back pain, it was obvious that it was being aggravated by her body weight. With her body insulated by well over one hundred pounds of excess body fat, it seemed unlikely that manipulation or physical therapy would have much effect in relieving the painful strain on her sensitive spinal joints. X-ray examination would be difficult because of her girth.

"Please don't tell me I'm too fat," Wanda pleaded. "I know I'm too fat. All I want is something for my back pain. I've been dieting off and on all my life, and it hasn't helped a bit."

There wasn't much I could do for Wanda but tell her that she needed to lose at least a hundred pounds of the extra fat she was carrying around. But rather than give her a printed diet sheet to follow, I tried to tell her how to eat properly. I told her about the high-fiber natural carbohydrate diet I recommend, and I gave her a list of the basic rules outlined in this chapter.

Dieting Can Make You Fat!

There is now evidence to indicate that extreme, low-calorie dieting might actually encourage the body to store fat. Apparently, rapid loss of body fat, which occurs during a "starvation diet," triggers a survival mechanism that conserves fuel so that the body can sustain itself with less food. There may even be a drop in resting metabolism along with increased efficiency in the consumption of energy. When the body loses 10 percent of its weight, for example, it may compensate by burning 15 percent fewer calories than normal. In the interest of self-preservation, the body simply responds to signals that a famine is imminent, adjusting its energy mechanism accordingly.

We all know that you cannot stay on a low-calorie, rapid-weight-loss diet for very long. When you switch back to normal eating, your body has become so efficient at conserving fuel (fat) that it begins to store more fat than ever in order to prepare for the next time that adequate food is not available.

When your body has regained the fat you lost, chances are you'll go on another starvation diet. Each time you resume normal eating, however, you regain a little more fat than before, until you finally lose the battle. You end up weighing more than you did when you first started dieting. Worst of all, each time you go on a diet that's too low in calories, you lose precious protein from your muscles and your organs. You regain the fat you lost, but not the muscle.

The up-and-down weight gain and loss resulting from this type of yo-yo dieting tends to promote a build-up of body fat at the expense of body protein, converting the body into a weak, flabby glob that's bound to weaken your back.

So what's the answer?

I would tell you what I told Wanda: Don't go on any diet that supplies less than 1,200 calories a day. Be sure to eat a variety of fresh, natural, high-fiber, low-fat foods that have been prepared without fat, sugar, oil, or white flour. Exercise regularly and eat three modest meals a day.

Healthy Diets and Calorie Reduction

If you are healthy and active and haven't conditioned your body's defensive mechanism with a starvation diet, you should be able to lose excess body fat on a diet that supplies 1,500 or more calories a day. Until your body has been reconditioned to normal food consumption, however, you may have to limit your energy intake to 1,200 to 1,500 calories a day. If you eat strictly *natural* foods, with emphasis on high-fiber carbohydrates, you'll find that it takes a lot of food to supply 1,200 calories. (See the 1,200-calorie diet at the end of this chapter.)

Even if you don't feel that you're losing weight on 1,200 calories a day, stick to the diet until your appetite mechanism regains control and your body metabolism is readjusted to normal eating. Then, you'll begin to lose a pound or two a week. And instead of reaching the plateau experienced by low-calorie dieters, you'll continue to lose more and more weight as your body normalizes its function and its reaction to food. Best of all, if you continue to eat properly, you can continue to eat normally and your body will automatically maintain a body weight that's best for you. Never again will you have to cut back to a dangerously low calorie intake.

How Wanda T. Finally Shed Her Excess Body Fat

Once Wanda learned how to eat properly, she began to lose weight slowly but surely. As her body weight lightened and her muscles grew stronger, she began to do some of the exercises described in Chapter 7. Weight loss became more rapid as Wanda became more active.

After several months, Wanda had lost most of her excess body fat. When she reached a "pleasingly plump" level, her back trouble disappeared. "During all the years I was carrying around that load of fat," Wanda recalled, "I spent so much of my time nursing my back that I could not care for my children properly. It's such a relief to get rid of the fat and the back pain that I feel like a new person. I sure look a lot better, and for the first time in years I feel good about myself."

If Wanda can do it, you can too. So read on.

The Health Bonuses of Proper Eating

This chapter has more to offer than cosmetic improvement and relief from backache. If you're overweight and you have back trouble, reducing your weight to relieve the strain on your back will make you, like Wanda, look better and feel better. The high-fiber, low-fat natural foods diet I advocate will also improve your health. It will help prevent colon cancer, heart disease, stroke, diabetes, and other diseases. Even if you aren't overweight, you should study this chapter carefully.

Get Rid of Backache by Getting Rid of Your Potbelly

You may be able to *prevent* the development or aggravation of back trouble by keeping your body weight light and balanced. The heavier you are, the more compression there is on the discs or cushions in the lower part of your spine. If your weight increases from 120 pounds to 200 pounds, for example, the pressure on your lumbar discs increases from 70 pounds to 120 pounds. If some of this weight is in the form of a big potbelly, the pressure on your lower back will be even greater. Protrusion of your abdomen in front will force you to lean backward in order to balance your body weight, increasing the leverage on your spine.

The bigger your potbelly and the farther out front it is, the greater the leverage on your spine. If you have ten pounds of potbelly centered 10 inches out in front of your spine, your back muscles must exert a force of 50 pounds to counterbalance the extra weight. This increases the pressure on your lower back by 50 extra pounds! Just imagine what a strain there is on the muscles and joints of the lower spine in an obese person who is carrying around a potbelly as big as a watermelon.

Don't let that happen to you. For cosmetic reasons as well as for back care, you should not carry around the "dead weight" of a potbelly.

Since exercise is important in preventing the development of a potbelly, even if you aren't overweight, be sure to do some of the abdominal exercises described in Chapter 7. If you are overweight, exercise will speed weight loss by forcing your body to burn stored fat for energy. The metabolic effects of regular exercise, in tearing down and building up muscle tissue, especially resistive exercise for the major muscle groups, will continue to burn calories after exercising, burning many more calories than those expended during the actual exercise. I keep my muscles developed by lifting weights in a half-hour workout two or three times a week. Although I spend a total of only one or two hours a week exercising, it seems that I can eat all I want without building up body fat. As long as my muscles are well developed and I exercise regularly, my calorie output during rest prevents the storage of calories supplied by a generous diet of fresh, natural foods.

Including back exercises in your reducing program will improve support for your spine while burning off body fat.

Note: The 1995 *Dietary Guidelines for Americans* (fourth edition) recommends that reducing diets be accompanied by thirty minutes or more of moderate physical activity—such as brisk walking, swimming, cycling, or pulling your own golf cart—every day.

Once your ideal weight has been reached, you must balance your physical activity with your food intake to prevent further weight gain or loss.

Other than some additional emphasis on use of exercise for weight control, the new 2000 *Dietary Guidelines* (fifth edition) has not changed much since its first edition in 1980. The guidelines continue to recommend consumption of a variety of grains, fruits, and vegetables, with a low intake of salt, sugar, saturated fat, and cholesterol.

The New High-Fiber, High-Carbohydrate Reducing Diet

In the past, most reducing diets advocated foods rich in protein and low in carbohydrate. Some popular "reducing" diets even allowed you to eat all the fat you wanted if you reduced your intake of carbohydrate to zero or a few grams. All of these diets proved to be harmful to health. Steer clear of fad low-carbohydrate, high-fat diets!

Today, most medically approved food plans are still based on the general rules outlined in the second edition of *Dietary Goals for the United States*, published in December of 1977 and updated as *Dietary Guidelines*. In this approach to eating, the emphasis is on carbohydrates, with about 58 percent of energy intake coming from carbohydrate, 12 percent from protein, and about 30 percent from fat. On a reducing diet that supplies less than 2,000 calories a day, however, about 20 percent of energy intake should probably come from protein in order to ensure that the diet supplies at least 60 grams of protein a day. Since animal protein also supplies fat, you will usually get adequate fat, even if you trim away all visible fat and avoid the use of cooking oils. Remember that whole-grain products, nuts, and some vegetables contain oil.

If you eliminate sugar and white-flour products from your diet and get your carbohydrates from fresh fruits, vegetables, and whole-grain products, the carbohydrates you consume will be high in fiber and low in calories, allowing consumption of a large volume of food. Natural complex carbohydrates are, in fact, much less fattening than the more concentrated proteins and fats.

How to Balance Your Diet

One of the best ways to assure a proper balance between carbohydrates, proteins, and fats without measuring grams and calories is to make food selections from all the basic food groups each day. In order to make sure that the greater part of your energy intake comes from carbohydrates, you should choose from six food groups rather than from the old four groups. In the four groups, fruits and vegetables were combined into one group, which tended to have the effect of encouraging an increased intake of meat and dairy products (which occupied two groups).

If you select something from each of the six food groups I recommend each day, you'll automatically get 50 to 60 percent of your energy from *natural* carbohydrates, since four of the groups supply fruits, vegetables, and whole-grain products.

Here are the six food groups from which daily food selections should be made:

1. Green and yellow vegetables (two or more servings)

2. Citrus fruits, tomatoes, and raw cabbage (two or more servings)

3. Potatoes, brown rice, and other vegetables and fruits (one or more servings)

4. Whole-grain bread, cereal, and flour (four or more servings)

5. Skimmed milk and skimmed milk products (two or more servings)

6. Lean meat, fish, eggs, skinned poultry, and dried peas and beans (two or more servings)

Selection of foods from all six food groups would ordinarily assure an adequate intake of vitamins and minerals. If you are on a reducing diet that supplies less than 2,000 calories a day, however, you should probably take a multiple vitamin-mineral supplement each day.

Foods in the protein and carbohydrate categories are never pure protein or pure carbohydrate. Meats, which are primarily protein, are often rich in saturated fat. Carbohydrate-rich grains and vegetables supply important unsaturated fat (essential fatty acids) as well as some protein. Remember that unsaturated fat in the diet should outweigh saturated fat two to one. If you make food selections from the six food groups, you won't be getting all your fat and protein from animal products. You'll get all the unsaturated fat you need from vegetables and whole-grain products. Combining grains and vegetables (such as rice and beans) will contribute some complete protein to your diet. The key is balanced variety.

Since too much fat of any kind may contribute to the development of cancer as well as to weight gain, it's important to keep the intake of all types of fat to a minimum. Remember that the saturated fat supplied by animal products tends to clog arteries, while the unsaturated fat supplied by vegetables and grains (and fish) tends to keep arteries open. Cholesterol, which has been implicated in the development of heart disease, is associated with animal fat and is not found in vegetable fats. Obviously, while you should keep your fat intake as low as possible, most of your fat should come from vegetables and whole-grain products in a predominantly carbohydrate diet.

The New Food Pyramid

In May of 1992, fifteen years after *Dietary Goals* reported that 58 percent of daily calorie intake should come from carbohydrates, the U.S. Department of Agriculture revised the four basic food groups into six groups in a pyramid fashion with four levels.

The base of the pyramid listed bread, rice, cereal, and pasta, recommending six to eleven servings. Next to the bottom level were vegetables, three to five servings, and fruits, two to four servings. The level next to the top listed milk, yogurt, and cheese, two to three servings, and meat, poultry, fish, dried beans, eggs, and nuts, two to three servings. At the top of the pyramid were fats and oils, to be used sparingly.

The purpose of rearranging the food groups, as suggested by the shape of the pyramid, was to increase carbohydrate intake and reduce fat intake.

It's important to remember, however, that your carbohydrate intake should consist of *natural* carbohydrates. Bread, cereal, and pasta should be of the whole-grain variety whenever possible. Rice should be brown and unpolished. Fruits should be fresh and raw. Vegetables should be prepared without grease or oil when they aren't eaten raw.

For adults, milk should be skimmed of fat, and yogurt should be of the low-fat variety with active culture.

If you use low-fat milk products, trim fat from meat, remove skin from poultry, and cook without fats or oils, you'll still get all the fat you need from the natural fat content of meats, nuts, and whole grains—and you'll be more successful with your reducing diet. If you make your food selections from the six groups outlined earlier, you'll automatically get the largest part of your calorie intake from natural carbohydrates with a minimum intake of fat. Try to make sure that at least two-thirds of what you consume for lunch and dinner contains foods of plant origin.

The Healthful Benefits of Fiber Supplied by Natural Carbohydrates

The fiber supplied by fresh fruits, vegetables, and whole-grain products is an important benefit of high-carbohydrate dieting. In addition to providing bulk that's low in calories, natural carbohydrates contain different kinds of fiber that convey different health benefits. The bran in whole-grain products helps prevent constipation, colon cancer, and diverticulosis by keeping the contents of the colon moist and bulky for easy elimination. The pectin supplied by the fiber of fruits and some vegetables helps lower blood cholesterol and keeps blood sugar under control. The lignin and the cellulose found in cereals and bran help slow absorption of calories.

Fiber in the bowel, particularly from oatmeal and apples, encourages the growth of friendly bacteria, which crowd out toxin-producing, unfriendly bacteria. Some forms of fiber, such as pectin, lignin, and gums, actually combine with toxins in the intestinal tract so that they can be eliminated in the stool.

While you need plenty of fiber in your diet, too much of one kind can have a harmful effect. An excessive amount of phytate-containing fiber supplied by whole-grain products might interfere with absorption of zinc, iron, calcium, and magnesium. Too much pectin supplied by fruits might interfere with absorption of vitamin B-12, and so on.

The best way to be assured of getting adequate and balanced amounts of different fibers is to eat a variety of fresh, natural foods from all the basic food groups. Stay away from one-food diets. Remember that while you're reducing your body weight to ease the strain on your back, you must protect your health by eating properly. It's not enough to lose weight simply by cutting your calorie intake or by eliminating foods. Limiting food selections to only a few foods in a low-calorie diet is courting disaster.

BEWARE OF FAD DIETS!

Although the U.S. Dietary Goals were formulated over twenty years ago, the recommendation that 48 percent of calorie intake should come from natural complex carbohydrates (fruits, vegetables, and whole grains) and 30 percent from fat is still valid. Any diet in which there is reduced calorie intake (including faddish high-protein or high-fat diets) can result in weight loss. But it is the consensus of experts that a diet that is predominately protein or fat can overload your kidneys, weaken your bones, trigger gout, raise blood fat, and cause imbalances that may lead to heart disease, cancer, and other diseases that shorten life. So don't fall prey to faddish eat-all-the-protein-and-fat-you-want diets. Moderation and variety with emphasis on fresh fruits, vegetables, and whole grains, along with a reduction in calorie intake, is the key to healthy eating and ideal body weight.

Basic Rules for Losing Weight

Before discussing how many calories you should consume each day to lose weight or to maintain your ideal body weight, there are some basic rules you should follow in molding your eating habits. Many people find that they can lose weight simply by observing these rules, without actually counting calories or measuring food portions. If you're not inclined to follow a specific diet plan, try following these four basic rules for a few weeks and see what happens.

1. **Try not to eat foods containing sugar or white flour.** One teaspoon of sugar contains only about 15 calories. A small amount of sugar is not going to hurt you. Unfortunately, the average American consumes far too much sugar—about 120 pounds a year! One reason for this high sugar consumption is that many of the canned and processed foods we eat contain

hidden sugar. Most canned foods, for example, contain sugar. One tablespoonful of catsup contains about one teaspoonful of sugar. A cola might contain 10 teaspoonfuls of sugar!

Obviously, while you should try to eliminate such sugar-sweetened foods as candy, cakes, pies, soft drinks, and refined cereals, you should make a special effort to substitute fresh, natural foods for canned, packaged, and refined or processed foods. You can sweeten whole-grain cereals with fresh or dried fruit. Honey is a good sweetener for hot cereal. Since honey is actually sweeter than sugar, you won't use as much honey as you would sugar.

White flour, like sugar, is a refined carbohydrate and can be just as fattening as sugar. Unlike whole-wheat flour, which is rich in fiber and nutrients, white flour contains no fiber and is more easily absorbed. The fiber in whole-grain flour *reduces* absorption of calories and provides bulk for your bowels. When you buy bread and other flour products, try to make sure that they are of the whole-grain variety. "Wheat flour" is actually white flour. Always select bread made from "whole wheat flour" rather than from "wheat flour." Remember that the more fiber breads and flours contain, the less fattening they are. And the coarser the product, the better for your health.

2. **Eat fish, skinned poultry, fresh fruits and vegetables, whole-grain breads and cereals, and cottage cheese and yogurt made from skimmed milk.** If you eat these natural foods instead of canned, refined, or processed foods, your calorie intake will be lower and your nutrient and fiber intake higher. Always cut away visible meat fat, and remove the skin from poultry. Remember, however, that some lean red meats may contain as much as 40 percent fat. So try to get most of your protein from fish and poultry.

Avoid lunchmeats, powdered potatoes, and other highly processed foods. If you use peanut butter as a source of protein, buy pure peanut butter from a health food store (now available in some grocery stores) and skim off the surface oil. The hydrogenated variety of peanut butter found in most grocery stores may contain sugar, preservatives, and other additives, along with a high percentage of saturated fat.

You can use lemon juice and vinegar on vegetable salads. Low-fat yogurt makes a good dressing for a baked potato.

3. **Use skimmed milk, vegetable juice, and water as beverages.** You should have at least one pint of milk—or its equivalent in milk products—each day to assure an adequate intake of calcium. Two cups (one pint) of milk will supply half your daily calcium requirement.

Since vegetable juices are lower in calories than fruit juice, it's always best to use vegetable juice rather than fruit juice for a beverage. With the exception of a morning glass of fruit juice for breakfast, you should always eat the whole fruit rather than squeeze it for juice. The pulp of fruit provides pectin and other important fibers that are beneficial to health. Besides, the pulp of fruit provides filling, low-calorie bulk as opposed to more concentrated, higher-calorie fruit juice.

When you are thirsty, especially after exercising, you should drink *water* rather than coffee, tea, or colas. Don't get into the habit of satisfying your thirst with soft drinks. Artificial beverages (made with manufactured ingredients) are not good for you, whether they're sweetened with sugar or with artificial sweeteners.

4. **Do not use fats or oils in cooking.** Since fats and oils contain more calories than any other food substance, you should avoid them whenever possible. You certainly should not add them to the foods you cook. You can steam vegetables, boil eggs, and broil or bake meat, poultry, or fish without using cooking oils. Instead of using meat fat as a seasoning for vegetables, you can use a bouillon cube. There isn't any natural food that cannot be cooked without fat or oil.

You already know that an excessive amount of fat in the diet can contribute to the development of cancer, hardening of the arteries, and other diseases. When you overheat fat or oil, fatty acids are broken down into a carcinogenic substance that can cause diarrhea by irritating the intestinal tract. If you do fry foods occasionally, use vegetable oil and keep heat low enough to avoid making the oil smoke.

Note: When calorie input permits, a little heart-friendly unsaturated fat can be obtained from nuts and avocados or from vegetable oil or olive oil added to salads. A tablespoon of oil contains about 120 calories. You should avoid animal fats (sources of saturated fat and cholesterol) and hydrogenated or processed fats, such as magarine, which may contain harmful trans-fatty acids.

How Mervin P. Relieved His Back Pain by Following a Simple Diet Plan

Mervin P. was a pipe fitter who often spent months away from home on special jobs. When he developed recurring back pain that caused him to lose job assignments, he visited my office seeking help. In addition to a worn-out disc in his lower spine, Mervin was 80 pounds overweight— and most of it was in his lower abdomen. In fact, Mervin had such a huge belly that he leaned backward when he walked.

"You'll always have some back trouble from your degenerated disc," I told Mervin. "But if you reduce your body weight and get rid of that potbelly, you'll get along a lot better."

But Mervin didn't want to go on a diet. "I can't follow a special diet," he argued. "I travel a lot, and I usually eat out."

Instead of giving Mervin a diet, I gave him some basic rules to follow—rules that would encourage him to eat properly while allowing him to select from foods available to him. When Mervin returned from a job six months later, he had lost a little over 40 pounds. His potbelly was gone, he was walking erect, and his back trouble was much improved.

"Since I got rid of that potbelly," Mervin reported happily, "I haven't had much back trouble. I followed those basic rules and lost weight without starving myself. Losing all that fat has practically cured my backache!"

A Sample Low-Fat, Low-Calorie Natural Foods Diet Plan

If you want to follow a few general rules so that you can avoid counting calories while reducing your body weight, try following this sample diet plan. *You can eat all the fresh vegetables you want* as long as they are prepared without sugar, grease, fat, or oil. (Throw out leftover bacon grease!) It's usually best to steam vegetables when they aren't eaten raw. Vegetables should be cooked only as long as necessary to soften them enough to permit penetration with a fork. When you cook a vegetable to a mush, you destroy fiber as well as nutrients.

Breakfast

One egg *or* a serving of lean ham, Canadian bacon, or veal.

One slice of whole-grain bread with a cup of skim milk *or* a whole-grain cereal with skim milk. (Cereal may be sweetened with fresh or dried fruit.)

One piece of citrus fruit *or* a glass of fruit juice.

Lunch

Fish *or* skinned chicken *or* a lean meat of your choice.

One dark green vegetable *or* one deep yellow vegetable.

One other vegetable of your choice.

One slice of whole-grain bread *or* a serving of corn bread.

One cup of vegetable juice, water, or skim milk as a beverage with meal.

For dessert: melon, fresh fruit, or dried fruit.

Dinner

A serving of the same meat dish you had at lunch *or* a serving of uncreamed cottage cheese, pot cheese, or farmer's cheese.

A fresh, raw vegetable salad laced with lemon juice.

A slice of whole-grain bread *or* a few whole-grain wafers.

A cup of vegetable juice *or* a cup of skim milk.

How Hannah B. Lost Weight on a Natural-Foods Diet Plan

Hannah wanted to know what types of foods to eat, but she did not want to count calories. "If you'll tell me what kind of foods to eat, I believe I can avoid overeating," she said.

Since Hannah had chronic backache caused by a spinal abnormality that was being aggravated by an overload of body fat, reducing her body weight was an important part of her treatment. So, I outlined a natural-foods diet plan especially for her. "Follow this vegetable-rich diet for at least a month before you decide whether it's working or not," I advised Hannah. "Even if weight loss is slow, the diet will improve your health."

After a few weeks on the diet, Hannah began to lose a pound or two a week. Eventually, she lost all of her excess body fat, and the result was a nearly pain-free back. "I'm pleased that my back is doing better," Hannah said, "but I'm even more pleased with the way I look."

How to Determine Your Calorie Requirement

If you follow the type of natural-foods diet plan I have just outlined, and stick with it for several weeks, you should be able to shed excess body fat without measuring your calorie intake. If you want complete control over your weight loss, however, so that you can eat as much as you possibly can and still lose a certain amount of weight, you should have a basic knowledge of calorie counting.

Generally, the average moderately active person must take in about 15 calories for each pound of ideal body weight each day in order to *maintain* that weight. A less active person might need only 12 calories per pound of ideal weight, while persons who work hard might need as many as 18 calories per pound. When more calories are taken in than the body can use, the excess calories are stored as fat.

The average person burns from 2,500 to 3,000 calories a day. A sedentary person might need only 2,500 calories a day, while a person engaged in manual labor might need as many as 5,000 calories a day. Even if you don't do anything but sit all day, your body needs about 1,500 calories a day to carry on its basic functions. Respiratory action, digestion, contraction of the heart muscle, and body metabolism, for example, burn calories. Such basic requirements are measured as the basal metabolic rate (BMR). The average man's BMR consumes about 1,650 calories, while a woman's basic functions consume about 1,350 calories. Since the basal metabolic rate declines with age, you need fewer calories as you grow older.

Calories and Your Ideal Weight

Before you can cut your calorie intake down to a safe level, you'll have to determine how many calories you should be taking in to maintain your *ideal* weight. You can find your ideal weight on a height-weight chart for men and women. Or, if you are a man, you may estimate your ideal weight simply by beginning with a base weight of 106 pounds and adding 5 pounds for each inch over 5 feet of height. If you are a woman, begin with a base weight of 100 pounds and add 5 pounds for each inch of height over 5 feet. For each inch under 5 feet, subtract 5 pounds.

Once you have estimated your ideal weight, you can estimate the number of calories you need to maintain that weight simply by multiplying the recommended number of calories per pound, usually about 15, depending upon how active you are.

How to Calculate Your Calorie Intake to Lose Weight

In order to force your body to burn stored fat as energy, you must take in fewer calories than you need to maintain your ideal weight. If you should and do weigh 150 pounds, for example, you would have to take in 2,250 calories a day to maintain that weight (150 pounds x 15 calories = 2,250 calories).

If you weigh 200 pounds and you should weight only 150 pounds, you would have to take in *less* than 2,250 calories a day in order to burn stored fat and lose weight. Since each pound of body fat contains about 3,500 calories, calorie intake would have to be reduced by 500 calories a day (cut to 1,750) to lose one pound of stored fat a week. (A 500-calorie deficit multiplied by seven days equals 3,500 calories, or one pound of fat.)

To lose *2 pounds* of fat a week in reaching an ideal weight of 150 pounds, you'd have to limit your calorie intake to 1,250, or 1,000 fewer calories than needed to maintain an ideal weight of 150 pounds. Remember that you are forcing your body to burn *stored* fat. This means that you must take in fewer calories than you burn each day. You cannot calculate your caloric need by estimating calories per pound and including inert, excess body fat. Your caloric need must be estimated according to requirements for maintaining ideal body weight, which would be closer to the actual number of calories you burn each day.

I've seen people who weigh 250 pounds estimate their calorie requirement to be 3,750 a day to maintain their existing weight, figuring 15 calories per pound of body weight. When they attempt to lose weight by reducing this estimated calorie requirement by 500 to 1,000 calories a day, their weight gain slows but they don't lose weight because they continue to exceed the actual number of calories they need to force burning of stored fat. Loss of stored fat will occur only when the number of calories burned each day exceeds the number taken in, which is best estimated by determining what your ideal weight should be. Otherwise, you simply continue to carry around stored fat that lies in reserve.

Note: If your body weight is light and you have only a few pounds of excess fat to lose, you may have to keep weight loss low and slow in order to keep your calorie intake above 1,200 calories. This might mean taking in each day only about 250 fewer calories than needed to maintain your estimated ideal body weight. You could lose muscle protein and develop a deficiency in essential nutrients when daily calorie intake drops below

1,200. It's always a good idea to take a multiple vitamin-mineral sup-plement when your diet supplies less than 2,000 calories a day.

WEIGHT RANGES FOR ADULTS

Height (without shoes)	Weight in pounds (without clothes)	
	19 to 34 years	35 years and over
5'0"	97–128	108–138
5'1"	101–132	111–143
5'2"	104–137	115–148
5'3"	107–141	119–152
5'4"	111–146	122–157
5'5"	114–150	126–162
5'6"	118–155	130–167
5'7"	121–160	134–172
5'8"	125–164	138–178
5'9"	129–169	142–183
5'10"	132–174	146–188
5'11"	136–179	151–194
6'0"	140–184	155–199
6'1"	144–189	159–205
6'2"	148–195	164–210
6'3"	152–200	168–216
6'4"	156–205	173–222
6'5"	160–211	177–228
6'6"	164–216	182–234

(Source: Diet and Health: Implications for Reducing Chronic Disease Risk, 1989, National Research Council, National Academy of Sciences.)

The higher weights in the ranges generally apply to men, who tend to have more muscle and bone; the lower weights more often apply to women, who have less muscle and bone.

Some newer weight charts evaluate body weight by using a "body mass index," or BMI. The chart assigns previously calculated numbers rang-ing from nineteen to forty to specific heights and weights, with any number over twenty-five indicating excessive weight. Body mass index is not very specific, however, and may not be accurate for bodybuilders and others who have unusual body structure. For most of us, the old height-weight charts, such as the one shown on the previous page, are adequate.

BODY MASS INDEX (BMI)

BMI	25	26	27	28	29	30	35	40
Ht.	Weight in pounds							
4'10"	119	124	129	134	138	143	167	191
4'11"	124	128	133	138	143	148	173	198
5'0"	128	133	138	143	148	153	179	204
5'1"	132	137	143	148	153	158	185	211
5'2"	136	142	147	153	158	164	191	218
5'3"	141	146	152	158	163	169	197	225
5'4"	145	151	152	163	169	174	204	232
5'5"	150	156	162	168	174	180	210	240
5'6"	155	161	167	173	179	186	216	247
5'7"	159	166	172	178	185	191	223	255
5'8"	164	171	177	184	190	197	230	262
5'9"	169	176	182	189	196	203	236	270
5'10"	174	181	188	195	202	207	243	278
5'11"	179	186	193	200	208	215	250	286
6'0"	184	191	199	206	213	221	258	294
6'1"	189	197	204	212	219	227	265	302
6'2"	194	202	210	218	225	233	272	311
6'3"	200	208	216	224	232	240	279	319
6'4"	205	213	221	230	238	246	287	328
	Overweight				Obese			

If your weight falls within the weight-height chart shown above, you may be overweight or obese, as indicated by the BMI numbers at the top of the chart. Many physicians prefer to use the body mass index as a method of estimating weight status.

How a Professor Cured His Backache by
Counting Calories

Unlike Wanda, Mervin, and Hannah, Dr. Norris S., an overweight college professor with a long history of chronic backache, wanted to calculate his calorie intake and measure his food portions. "I want to be able to control my weight loss as much as possible," he explained, "so that I can get the most out of my eating and my weight loss."

I told Dr. Norris how to determine the calorie requirement for his ideal weight and then how to measure and balance his energy intake from carbohydrates, proteins, and fats. For him, this approach worked best. After he lost from 1 to 2 pounds a week over a period of several months, his back trouble became a minor problem.

"After I lost 32 pounds," Norris observed, "I quit having acute back pain. I still have a little back trouble, but I haven't had to go to bed or take time off from work. Best of all, I haven't had to take any painkilling medication. Also, looking better has encouraged me to take a little exercise, which has made my back stronger."

Many back patients, like Norris, look so much better when excess body fat is reduced that they enthusiastically undertake a program of exercise to further improve their appearance. The result is such an improvement in the function of supporting back muscles that a lighter body weight supported by stronger muscles often "cures" back trouble.

How to Balance Energy Nutrients

A properly balanced 1,200-calorie diet with food selections from the six basic food groups listed earlier will automatically provide a good balance of carbohydrate, protein, and fat. Such a diet, with 1,200 calories, should supply about 576 carbohydrate calories, 264 protein calories, and 360 fat calories. Since one gram of carbohydrate contains four calories, 576 carbohydrate calories divided by four equal 144 grams of carbohydrate. One gram of protein also supplies four calories, so 264 protein calories divided by four equal 66 grams of protein. One gram of fat supplies *nine* calories, which means that 360 fat calories are equal to only 40 grams of fat. Once you know the number of calories supplied by the gram weights of the carbohydrate, protein, and fat you consume, you can calculate the percentage of calories you obtain from these food types. A twelve hundred-calorie diet, for example, that contains 144 grams of carbohydrate supplying 576

6

calories means that 48 percent of your calorie intake is from carbohydrate, which is the recommended level. For a comprehensive list of food values, see *Composition of Foods: Raw, Processed, Prepared* (Agriculture Handbook No. 8, U.S. Government Printing Office, Washington, DC).

Most of us will prefer to balance our diet simply by making food selections from all the basic food groups, with emphasis on fresh, natural carbohydrates.

Two Sample Balanced Calorie-Counting Reducing Diets

Here are a couple of low-calorie, calorie-counting diets that will meet the average person's needs for a reducing diet. If you are a female, or if you are a small person, the 1,200-plus-calorie diet may be best. Males, or persons with large frames, may fare better on the 1,500-plus-calorie diet.

Remember that these are sample diets that allow you to choose the foods you like best, of certain types, but with restrictions on quantity. If you eliminate sugar and white flour products, which are highly concentrated in calories, and stick to fresh, natural foods with up to 60 percent of your calories coming from natural carbohydrates, you'll find that both plans will provide plenty of food. If you feel that your stomach is not full enough, you can drink a glass of water before or after each meal or you may drink a cup of bouillon between meals. You may also snack on raw vegetables. Plain yogurt makes a good low-calorie dip.

A 1,200-PLUS–CALORIE DIET

Breakfast

1 piece fresh fruit

1 slice whole-grain bread topped with one egg *or* 1 serving of whole-grain cereal mixed with 1 tablespoonful of miller's bran

1 cup skim milk

Unsweetened coffee or tea if desired

Note: You may alternate the egg and the cereal so that you have 3 eggs a week.

Lunch

3 ounces chicken or fish

½ cup cooked vegetable

Green salad with vinegar or lemon juice dressing

1 slice whole-grain bread

1 piece fresh fruit

Water or unsweetened tea

Dinner

4 ounces chicken or fish

2 cooked vegetables, ½ cup each

or

1 cooked vegetable and a raw salad

1 slice whole-grain bread

1 piece fresh fruit

Water (with lemon or lime juice if desired) or vegetable juice

Bedtime snack

1 cup skim milk or 1–2 cup cottage cheese with 1 piece fresh fruit

A 1,500-PLUS–CALORIE DIET

Breakfast

6 ounces fruit juice

1 serving whole-grain cereal with diced fruit

or

1 slice whole-grain bread topped with one egg and 1 slice whole-grain bread with 1 pat of butter

1 piece fresh fruit

1 cup skim milk

Unsweetened coffee if desired

Lunch

3 ounces lean meat, chicken, or fish

2 cooked vegetables, ½ cup each

Green salad with lemon juice dressing

2 slices whole-grain bread

1 piece fresh fruit

Water or unsweetened tea, with lemon if desired

Dinner

3 ounces lean meat, chicken, or fish

2 cooked vegetables, ½ cup each

Green salad with vinegar or lemon juice dressing

2 slices whole-grain bread

1 piece fresh fruit

Water or vegetable juice

Bedtime snack

1 cup skim milk or 1 ounce hard cheese

1 slice whole-grain bread

Note: Fruit allowed with meals can be reserved for between-meal snacks if desired.

How Adelaide R. Ate Her Backache Away

Adelaide R. relieved her backache by losing 59 pounds on a 1,200 to 1,500 calorie diet. In the process, she became sold on the healthful benefits of eating natural foods. "I lost nearly 30 pounds in only a few months," she said, "and I had plenty to eat. I never knew that you could eat so much and lose weight. I intend to keep eating fresh, natural foods from now on, even if I never have another backache."

You Can Eat Heartily with Natural Foods!

When a diet consists of low-fat natural foods that are prepared without sugar, grease, fat, or oil, the amount of food needed to supply 1,500 or more calories might be more than some people can eat. But remember that you must include some of all the basic foods in order to meet the nutritional requirements of your body. You need at least the equivalent of two cups of milk each day, along with other foods that supply calcium, to keep your bones strong, especially your vertebrae. So don't try to substitute high-calorie refined foods for some of your less favorite natural foods.

Don't worry about the apparent absence of fat in your diet. You need only about fifteen to twenty-five grams of dietary fat daily to provide essential fatty acids and to serve as a carrier for fat-soluble vitamins. Otherwise, there is no specific requirement for fat as a nutrient in your diet. Lean meats and grains will supply all the fats and oils you need. Seeds and nuts are especially rich in fat.

What About Alcohol?

According to the December, 1995, fourth edition of the U.S. Department of Agriculture's *Dietary Guidelines for Americans,* "moderate" use of alcohol with meals may lower risk of coronary heart disease in some individuals and is permissible for some adults. Moderation is defined as no more than one drink per day for women who are not pregnant and no more than two drinks per day for men.

Remember, however, that alcoholic beverages supply 7 calories per gram with few or no nutrients. Natural carbohydrates, which are loaded with vitamins and minerals, supply only 4 calories per gram.

The Selection and Preparation of Foods Is Important

The first thing you must do when selecting foods is to make sure that the foods agree with you as well as meet your needs. If the lactose in fresh milk disturbs your intestinal tract, you may have to switch to fermented milk products in which lactose has been converted to lactic acid. If you have intestinal problems that have been traced to the gluten in wheat, rye, oats, and barley, you'll have to avoid all grains except corn and rice. Vegetarians can get the protein and the vitamin B-12 they need from other foods. Combinations of rice and beans, for example, or peanut butter on whole-grain bread, can supply complete protein. Eggs and milk products can supply vitamin B-12 as well as protein.

No one food is indispensable. If you don't like one particular vegetable or fruit, you can substitute another. There are a variety of whole-grain products to choose from. You can eat chicken or fish rather than beef or pork. But remember that seafood supplies important iodine. If you choose not to eat red meats, which are rich in iron, you should make a special effort to eat iron-rich dried fruits, legumes, and whole-grain products.

Try to avoid eliminating any wholesome, natural food from your reducing diet. Eat a variety of foods from all the basic food groups every day.

To Cook or Not to Cook

On a low-calorie diet, it's essential that the foods you select be properly prepared to conserve nutrients. Vegetables should be cooked with as little heat and water as possible in order to prevent loss of heat-sensitive and water-soluble vitamins and to avoid destruction of fiber. Fruits should always be eaten raw. When fruits and vegetables are cooked to a mush, destruction of the fiber makes them more digestible, thus more fattening.

While vegetables should be cooked as little as possible, meats should always be thoroughly cooked in order to kill parasites. I recommend that you order beef and pork well-done. You should never eat pink poultry or rare ground meat, lest you be poisoned by E. coli or salmonella bacteria.

Remember to cut away all visible fat from your meats and to peel the skin from poultry. Bake, broil, barbecue, or stew your meats. You may cook meats any way you like as long as you don't batter or fry them. The less animal fat you consume, the better.

Eggs are best boiled, poached, or scrambled. You shouldn't eat raw eggs, since they contain a substance (avidin) that might interfere with absorption of the B vitamin biotin. Besides, a raw egg might be contaminated with disease-producing bacteria.

You already know that the best way to cook a vegetable is to steam it a little. When you boil a vegetable, the only seasoning you might need is a little salt or a bouillon cube. Use of microwaves is a good, quick way to cook vegetables. When you microwave a vegetable in a teaspoon of water, it will retain more vitamins than it would if it were cooked on a stove.

It's usually best to bake potatoes in their skins. Frying a potato increases its calorie content tremendously. Potato chips, for example, are 40 percent fat compared to 0.1 percent fat in a baked potato. When a potato is fried with its skin, it might actually be slightly toxic. (Glycoalkaloids, a natural toxic substance found in potato skins, are more concentrated in fried skins. Sprouted, green, or dried potatoes may contain toxic levels of glycoalkaloids. *You should always peel sprouted or green potatoes.*)

A medium size potato contains only about 100 calories and is very nutritious. Baked potatoes and milk together supply some of all the essential nutrients. Don't hesitate to include baked potatoes in a reducing diet.

Cook One Day at a Time

Cook your vegetables fresh each day so that nutrients won't be lost to storage and reheating. Whenever possible, select produce that is garden fresh. Fruits and vegetables lose nutrients when they are stored for shipping and distribution.

Remember that on a low-calorie diet your nutrient intake may also be reduced. You cannot afford to lose nutrients to improper cooking methods or to prolonged storage. You need all the micronutrients that fresh food can supply to keep your muscles and bones strong and healthy and to protect your back.

SUMMARY

1. Excessive body weight can aggravate lower back trouble by increasing pressure on joints and discs.

2. A potbelly multiplies the stress on your spine by placing muscle-straining leverage on your lower back.

3. Modern dieting methods stress a greater intake of carbohydrates, with about 60 percent of energy intake coming from fresh fruits, vegetables, and whole-grain products.

4. Selection of foods from the six basic food groups will assure a greater intake of fiber-rich carbohydrates.

5. It's never a good idea to go below 1,200 calories a day in an effort to reduce body fat.

6. Low-calorie "starvation diets" result in loss of valuable protein in muscles and organs.

7. Diets that supply less than 2,000 calories a day should be supplemented with multiple vitamins and minerals.

8. Your daily diet should supply the equivalent of two cups of milk in order to provide the calcium your body needs to keep your vertebrae strong.

9. Whenever possible, foods should be prepared without adding fat, oil, or white flour.

10. Whole grains and meats should always be thoroughly cooked; vegetables should be cooked only slightly, and fruits should be eaten raw.

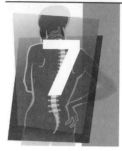

Protective and Remedial Exercise in a Personalized Back-Care Program

Wesley R. was a former college football player and weightlifter. When he graduated from college, he continued to visit the gym to do a little weightlifting. But after a few years, he gradually slipped into a more sedentary life, spending most of his time riding in his automobile on company business. Although Wesley felt that he was "staying in shape," he was exercising only about once a week. And he was doing less and less with each passing month.

Despite a gradual buildup of body fat, Wesley still visualized himself as the fit, lean athlete he was as a college senior. So it wasn't surprising that he occasionally attempted to duplicate some of the feats he performed in days gone by.

One holiday weekend, Wesley undertook the task of cutting down a dead pine tree. While he was loading the tree sections onto a truck, he felt a sharp pain in his lower back. A few hours later, he was unable to walk. The slightest movement caused excruciating pain and muscle spasm.

When I told Wesley that he had probably strained his back, he disagreed. "There must be something else wrong, Doc," he argued. "I'm too strong to strain my back. When I was in college, I could deadlift 500 pounds."

Like many of us, Wesley could not see the gradual deterioration that was taking place in his body. It never occurred to him that he was not the same man he was in college. Combining improper lifting techniques with weak back muscles was more than enough to pull the muscles in his back.

It took Wesley several weeks to recover from his injury. When he finally did go back to work, he had been replaced as district manager. "You've got to help me get back in shape," Wesley pleaded. "I'm scared to death that I'll hurt my back again—and I cannot afford to lose another job."

I instructed Wesley in many of the exercises described in this chapter. "No matter how strong you may become," I warned Wesley, "you'll always have to be careful about how you lift. Strong muscles are not going to protect your spine if you don't know how to lift properly."

Luckily, Wesley was able to avoid further injury. After a few months of exercising, his back muscles were considerably stronger. When I ran into him a few years later, he looked strong and fit.

"Your exercise program did wonders for me," Wesley reported. "I'm still doing it. I'm also going to the gym a couple of times a week to lift weights. But don't worry. I'm taking care to lift properly to avoid straining my back."

Exercise Is an Important Preventive Measure

Many backache specialists feel that exercise is the single most important measure to be taken for preventing backache. Some feel that good posture is most important. You already know from reading the chapter on weight control that weak abdominal muscles allow the development of a potbelly that places an off-balance strain on the spine, contributing to swayback and other problems.

There are 434 muscles in the body, accounting for about one-half of the total body weight. Lack of full-body exercise results in sagging, flabby muscles that may fail to support and protect the spine adequately in everyday activities. Simple postural strains then become a big problem. The muscles and joints of the back are easily strained with only moderate exertion. Heavy exertion and awkward movements may force shifting of loads from weak muscles to ligaments, resulting in a painful joint strain.

While it's important to lift properly to protect a weak back, it's just as important to lift properly to protect a strong back. So be sure to read Chapter 9 for instructions on correct lifting techniques.

Muscles Should Have Reserve Strength

When back muscles are properly strengthened, they have enough strength to perform daily duties without overtaxing your muscles or your spine.

For exercise to be effective in protecting your spine, muscles must be evenly developed on all sides of your trunk so that they hold your spine erect—much like the guy wires that support a radio tower. Strong back muscles won't protect your spine adequately if your abdominal muscles are weak. You must be strong in front as well as in back.

Unfortunately, most exercises tend to develop the muscles on the back of the spine. Even when a person does not take regular exercise, the back muscles get a certain amount of exercise in everyday activities. Thus, most of the time, it's the *abdominal* muscles and not the back muscles that are weakest.

Many exercise programs prescribed by doctors are often more of a stretching program than an exercise program. Many of the exercises call for passive forced flexion of the spine, as in toe touching. Such flexion-type exercises do not strengthen back muscles and might even place excessive compression on weak spinal discs. They might also overstretch tendons. One exercise in a popular set of exercises has the patient sit in a chair and lean forward, placing the head between the knees—something I would not recommend.

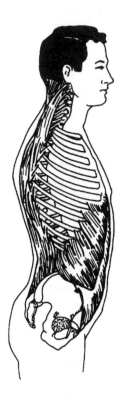

Figure 7-1. Muscles on both sides of the trunk are important for supporting the spine. A few simple basic exercises to strengthen back and abdominal muscles can do a lot to help prevent back trouble.

You'll learn in Chapter 9 that there is more pressure on your discs when you sit than when you stand. When you lean forward in a sitting position, the pressure on your discs is increased tremendously. Such exercises not only fail to strengthen your muscles but may actually do your spine more harm than good. So it's important that you select your back exercises carefully.

Special Benefits from Back Exercises

You'll learn in this chapter which exercises to do and how to do them properly. When they are evenly developed, your abdominal and back muscles will serve as a muscular corset that will support and protect your spine on all sides. Exercise will also strengthen your vertebrae, since the strength of bone increases in reaction to stress and pressure. You'll look better, too, since an improvement in muscle tone will lift up sagging tissues and flatten your abdomen. With any kind of regular exercise, you'll find it easier to keep your body lean and shapely.

For back exercises to be effective in building support for your spine, they must be specific. Some exercises are good for your back and some are bad. Bent-knee sit-ups, for example, will help protect your back by strengthening your hip flexors and your abdominal muscles. Straight-leg sit-ups, on the other hand, might strain your lower back by placing excessive leverage on your lumbar spine. If you have a specific back problem, your exercise program must be tailored to fit your needs.

As you study this chapter, you can select the exercises you need to do and avoid those that might aggravate your back trouble.

If you have back pain, go back to Chapter 4 and try the "Four Simple Back Exercises" described in that chapter. The exercises described in this chapter are designed to strengthen weak supporting muscles *after* your acute back pain has subsided. You'll find special stretching exercises in Chapter 5, along with passive movements that are designed to loosen and align your vertebrae.

How Sheila R. Achieved Permanent Relief from Backache by Exercising

Shelia R. had been experiencing recurring back trouble for years. Each day of twelve years as a bank teller ended with burning, aching back pain. "I've had back pain so long that I ought to be used to it by now," she said. "But my back hurts more now than ever before. I've even thought about applying for disability retirement, but my doctor cannot find anything wrong with my back."

When I saw Shelia in my office, she slumped and moved about like someone weakened by an extended illness. Her back muscles were flabby and inflamed. "Do you exercise?" I asked Shelia. "Heavens no," she responded. "I'm too tired and hurt too much at the end of the day to exercise."

It wasn't hard to figure out what Shelia's problem was. Inactivity combined with long hours of postural strain had allowed weakened muscles to become excessively fatigued and inflamed. The more inflamed her muscles became, the less active she became. Shelia had fallen into that vicious cycle of weakness, fatigue, and inactivity that leads to chronic backache, which is often diagnosed as fibromyositis or myofascitis. All she had to do to get permanent relief was to perform a few special exercises over a period of several weeks. By doing many of the exercises described in this chapter, Shelia was eventually able to complete a day without any backache at all.

"Regular exercise seems to have given me permanent relief from backache," Shelia reported after a couple of pain-free months. "I'm going to keep doing my exercises, and I'm going to make my husband do them too."

Begin Your Exercise Program with Abdominal Exercises

Since the abdominal muscles are often the weakest of the muscles supporting the spine, let's begin with a description of special abdominal exercises. No matter what type of back trouble you're having, you must strengthen your abdominal muscles—or at least keep them strong.

Select the exercises that are best suited for you. Don't do any exercise that causes pain. If you have had back surgery, see your doctor for special instructions.

Bent-Knee Sit-Ups

Your abdominal muscles and the hip flexors or psoas muscles that attach between your lumbar vertebrae and the top of your thigh bones provide support on the *front* of your spine. You can strengthen all these muscles by doing the common sit-up. You should always keep your knees bent when doing sit-ups, however, so that excessive leverage won't be placed on your hip-flexor muscles and your lumbar spine. You should also make sure that you tilt your pelvis so that your lower back is flat on the floor and not arched. This "pelvic tilt," which is easily achieved with the knees bent, greatly reduces the leverage on your lumbar spine.

If your abdominal muscles are too weak to do a sit-up, you can get assistance from your hip flexors by anchoring your feet under a heavy sofa. Some people with weak abdominal muscles may find that straight-leg sit-ups are easier to do than bent-knee sit-ups, especially with the feet anchored. Straightening the legs and anchoring the feet simply shifts most of the load from the abdominal muscles to the psoas muscles (hip flexors). Remember, also, that straight-leg sit-ups can place too much leverage on a weak lower spine. Furthermore, straight-leg sit-ups with the feet anchored might *overdevelop* the hip flexors, creating too much pull on the front of the spine. This might contribute to the development of swayback and other low-back problems.

Simply bending your knees during a sit-up will reduce the load on hip flexors by 70 percent, thus greatly reducing the pull on your lower spine. Obviously, bent-knee sit-ups are more specific for your abdominal muscles but will still provide some exercise for your hip flexors.

Holding your arms out in front (or on your chest) during a sit-up will make the exercise a little easier to do. But as you become stronger, you should place your hands behind your head in order to make the exercise more resistive.

Stretch Your Hip Flexors after Sit-ups

Since bent-knee sit-ups use your hip flexors in a shortened position, it might be a good idea to follow sit-ups with an exercise that's designed to *stretch* your hip flexors. Otherwise, shortening of your hip flexors might create enough of a pull to produce a swayback when you stand.

One good way to stretch your hip flexors without uncomfortable arching of your spine is to do a tripod leg-extension exercise. Get down on your hands and knees and then straighten one leg out, lifting it back and up as high as you can. This exercise will also strengthen gluteal (hip) and spina erecta (back) muscles without excessive extension (arching) of your lower back.

Abdominal Exercise the Easy Way

If you find bent-knee sit-ups too difficult to do, even with your feet anchored and your arms out in front, you can do a trunk curl or a half sit-up. Simply lie on your back with your arms at your sides and your knees bent and lift only your head and shoulders from the floor by curling your upper body, as in beginning a sit-up.

Once the trunk is curled and the abdominal muscles are contracted, the hip flexors take over in completing a sit-up. So it's not really necessary to complete a sit-up to exercise the abdominal muscles.

Strengthening Weak Hip Flexors

If a full sit-up is difficult to do with the feet anchored but does not cause pain, the problem might be weak hip flexors. When this is the case, the hip flexors should be strengthened by doing leg raises.

Lie flat on your back and raise one straight leg as high as you can. Exercise both sides equally. When you can do so without discomfort, raise both straight legs together. If this causes back pain, do bent-knee leg raises, bending your knees as necessary to eliminate pain or discomfort.

Begin doing bent-knee sit-ups when your hip flexors have strengthened and you are able to do so.

Frog kicks, or bent-knee leg lifts (with a trunk curl) while hanging from a chinning bar, combines spinal stretching with abdominal and hip-flexor exercise.

Take your time in an abdominal-strengthening program. When you are able to do fifteen or twenty bent-knee sit-ups, you can assume that your abdominal muscles and your hip flexors are strong enough to support your spine in front.

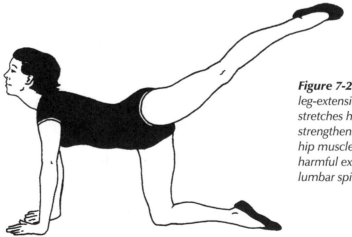

Figure 7-2. The tripod leg-extension exercise stretches hip flexors and strengthens back and hip muscles without harmful extension of the lumbar spine.

Strengthening the Supporting Muscles on the Back of Your Spine

The spina erecta muscles on the back of your spine are normally quite strong, since you use them in just about everything you do. The problem comes when you lift improperly, placing excessive leverage on your spine or when you overload your back muscles. Of course, the stronger your back muscles are, the less the chance that you might overload them in unaccustomed exertion. This is why you should strengthen your back muscles so they will be strong enough to handle emergencies and *more* than strong enough to perform daily tasks.

Other body muscles must also be strong enough to provide maximum protection for your back. When you lift a heavy weight, for example, you know that you should squat down and lift with your *legs*. If your legs are weak, there'll be a tendency to lift with your back by bending your hips rather than your knees.

Even when your back muscles are strong, you should never attempt to lift with your back instead of with your legs. If you should happen to have some structural instability in your lower spine, the leverage placed on your spine by the pull of strong back muscles might result in a severe joint or ligament strain.

You'll learn in Chapter 9 how to use your legs in lifting. In the meantime, remember that *all* the exercises described in this chapter, even the leg exercises, will provide important protection for your back.

Condition Your Back Muscles Gradually

During World War II, when I was a lad of about sixteen years of age, I took a job in a bowling alley setting up tenpins. In those days, pins were set manually, requiring the "pin boy" to jump down from his perch and bend over to replace the pins one at a time by hand. At the end of the first day, after several hours on the job, I developed such a severe backache that I walked back and forth in agony. My back muscles ached severely from unaccustomed exertion, even though I was in good physical shape. I learned from that experience that no matter how physically fit you might be, you must condition yourself for new activities, especially when back muscles are involved.

That was over fifty years ago. I still remember the agony I suffered when I see a patient with a similar backache. I feel a special obligation to do all I can to help my patients *prevent* such misery.

How Daniel R. Prevented Injury by Conditioning His Muscles

When Daniel R. visited my office complaining of lower back trouble, he informed me that he was planning to switch from selling insurance to driving and loading a truck. "You'd better begin an exercise program before you begin your new job," I warned Daniel, "or you might develop the worst backache you've ever had."

I recommended bent-knee sit-ups, a back-arching exercise, squats, and a couple of barbell exercises for Daniel. The result was that he began his new job without any back trouble whatsoever. "I breezed through the first few days as if I were an old pro," Daniel told me later. "Without the exercises, I'm sure I would have had some back trouble. Actually, I'm having *less* back trouble now than before, even though I'm working much harder."

No matter what type of work you do, you need to keep your back muscles strong. If you are a sedentary person and you are planning to begin a new job or some new physical activity requiring unaccustomed exertion, you should prepare your back muscles for the challenge by exercising them beforehand. Otherwise, you might suffer a severe backache or a damaging strain.

Developing Your Spina Erecta Muscles

The thick ridges of muscle running up and down each side of your spine are called spina erecta muscles. These muscles literally hold your spine erect, pulling you into an erect posture. There is constant tension in these muscles when you stand and walk. When back muscles are weak and flabby, simple postural strains can cause backache. When you lean forward to brush your teeth or to lift an object, the spina erecta muscles suspend your spine from top to bottom, using the base of your spine as a fulcrum. If your back muscles are weak, the joints and ligaments at the bottom of the spine may be forced to assume more than their share of the load.

Obviously, it's important to keep your back muscles strong in order to protect spinal joints and ligaments.

The Prone Back Arch

The simplest way to strengthen your spina erecta muscles is to do a back-arching exercise while lying face down. You can increase the range of motion of your spine without harm by doing the exercise from a cushion that supports your pelvis.

Lie face down with a sofa cushion under your pelvis and your feet anchored under the edge of a heavy sofa. Without using your arms, arch your upper body from the floor. Do not attempt to arch up as high as you

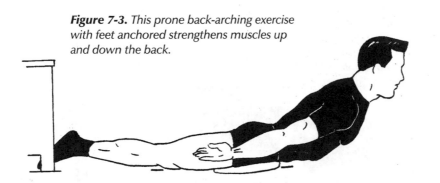

Figure 7-3. *This prone back-arching exercise with feet anchored strengthens muscles up and down the back.*

can. Stay well within a comfortable range of motion. Stop when you feel pain or discomfort.

Always warm up by doing a few repetitions and then rest a minute or two before doing a second set of the exercise. Work your way up to twelve to fifteen repetitions.

People with arthritis, osteoporosis, and other conditions that produce slumping of the spine should do this exercise regularly in order to keep the spine as straight as possible. Young people with epiphysitis or Scheuermann's disease (an inflammation that softens growth centers in the vertebrae, causing a slumping of the upper back) should make a special effort to do this exercise daily. Good posture is equally important, as you'll learn in Chapter 9.

Few back conditions will be aggravated by this back-arching exercise, but you should go by the way you feel. If the exercise causes you pain when you do it, stop!

The Prone One-Leg Raise

If you want to exercise your back muscles without uncomfortable hyperextension of your spine, try doing prone one-leg raises.

Lie face down and raise one straight leg as high as you can. Exercise both legs equally. Work up to twelve to fifteen repetitions with each leg.

The Supine Bridge

You can also strengthen your back and hip muscles with a safe, easy exercise by arching up from a supine position.

Lie on your back with your knees bent, your feet flat on the floor, and your arms at your sides (or on your abdomen). Lift your body from the floor

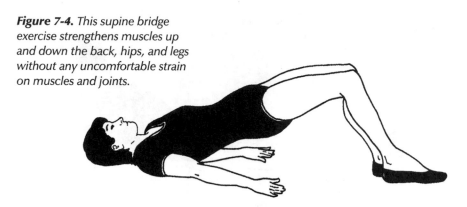

Figure 7-4. *This supine bridge exercise strengthens muscles up and down the back, hips, and legs without any uncomfortable strain on muscles and joints.*

so that your weight is supported only by your feet and your upper back to form a bridge. For additional resistance, you may hold a weight on your abdomen. Work up to twelve to fifteen repetitions. Be sure to support your weight with your upper back rather than with your head and neck. This exercise is not the same as a "wrestler's bridge."

Strengthen Your Legs to Protect Your Back

When **Edwin C.** injured his back for the third time lifting his grandchildren, I asked him if he could do a full squat. "Yes, I can," he replied. But when he squatted down, he could not come back up without leaning forward and placing his hands on his knees. It was obvious that Edwin's legs were too weak to squat down and lift a heavy object properly. Instead of lifting with his legs, he would lean forward and lift with his back.

Using the back in such a manner places a tremendous leverage on the muscles and joints of the lower spine. If there happens to be a defect or deformity in the lower joints of the spine, instability could result in a severely painful, crippling ligamentous strain. In any event, improper lifting techniques resulting from weak muscles are more likely to result in a lower back *joint* strain than a muscle strain. Repeated strains will further weaken the lower spine. Remember that a strain usually involves muscles and tendons, while a sprain, which is more serious, may involve stretching or tearing of joint ligaments. Back off when you feel that you may be straining your back.

I gave Edwin a set of exercises that included a squatting exercise. "When you are able to do at least a half dozen free, unassisted full squats," I told him, "you'll be able to use your legs in a correct lifting technique. Come back to see me in two months and let me know how you're doing."

When Edwin returned a few months later, he eagerly demonstrated his ability to squat with his trunk erect and his hands on his hips. "I sure feel stronger since I strengthened my legs," he stated emphatically while squatting repeatedly. "In addition to lifting better, I have more endurance, since everything I do now seems much easier."

The Proper Way to Squat

The best way to squat to strengthen your thighs is to squat with your heels on a board. This way, you can keep your spine vertical while squatting low.

Many people find it difficult to squat flat-footed without leaning forward, lest they topple over backward. The weaker the legs, the greater the tendency to lean forward, placing a greater strain on the lower back. Placing a board under the heels will reduce the tendency to lean forward while squatting. As your back and your legs become stronger from exercising, however, you should practice flat-footed squatting in order to further strengthen low-back, hip, and buttock muscles.

If you cannot do a full squat, start with *half* squats or hold a bedpost or other support for assistance. You can do a half squat simply by sitting in a chair and then standing up while keeping your spine as vertical as possible.

When you cannot squat because of arthritis or a knee injury, try to keep your thigh muscles strong by doing a leg-extension exercise. Just sit on a table with your lower legs dangling and lift a weight with your foot by locking your leg out straight.

Strengthen Your Entire Body

Overall body strength can be very important in protecting your back from strain. When you use your arms to push and pull, whether you're cleaning house or changing a tire on your automobile, there'll be less strain on your back if your arms and shoulders are strong. When your extremities are weak, you tend to lift more with your back than with your arms and your legs.

Any good overall body-strengthening program would be beneficial in building protection for your back. Simple resistive exercises such as push-ups, sit-ups, chins, and squats would be fine. Progressive resistance exercise with barbells and dumbbells might even be better, since you'll be doing controlled lifting exercises that can be made progressively more resistive as you grow stronger. Such basic barbell exercises as curls, presses, rowing motions, and squats can be done by anyone. Remember, however, that barbell exercises should be done to strengthen a weak back only when freedom from pain permits the use of such exercises. You should not lift weights while you are suffering from back pain.

When back pain is really acute, simply moving around can be difficult. Getting from your bed to the toilet or getting out of your car after a short trip can be an ordeal. Until you have recovered from back pain or a back injury, don't worry about doing muscle-strengthening exercises. It will be enough to move your joints through a full range of movement with simple bending exercises.

Strengthen Back Muscles with One Barbell Exercise

Simple bent-knee deadlifts with a barbell will provide good exercise for all of the muscles involved in lifting—from your shoulders to your legs. If performed properly, this exercise will also develop correct lifting techniques.

Squat down with your head up and your back as flat and as vertical as possible. Keep your back flat while lifting a barbell from the floor. At the completion of the lift, stand erect and lean backward a little while supporting the barbell down at arm's length in front.

Repeat the lift several times, keeping both feet flat on the floor while lifting. Be sure to squat low and keep your back flat so that you can lift with your legs. Be careful not to use more weight than you can handle comfortably for several repetitions.

Note: If you have low back or hip trouble, it might be a good idea to place each end of your barbell on a block or box that is up to two feet high. This will reduce squatting and flexion enough to decrease the leverage on your lower back, thus providing the mechanical advantage you need to avoid strain at the bottom of your spine.

I have a barbell in my backyard where I exercise about twice a week. I lift the barbell off two solid wooden blocks that are about 14 inches high. If you exercise in a gym, you can support the barbell on the supporting pins of a power rack at a level that suits you best.

What About Your Flank?

Generally, when you exercise your back muscles and your abdominal muscles, you'll develop adequate muscle support on all sides of your spine. But it won't hurt to do a little resistive side bending for a little extra strength on each side. The best way to do this is to bend from side to side while holding a dumbbell in one hand. Eight to ten repetitions comfortably performed with moderate resistance will do the job. Be sure to exercise both sides equally by holding the weight first in one hand and then in the other hand.

Twisting bent-knee sit-ups: Touching the right elbow to the left knee and then the left elbow to the right knee in succeeding repetitions will help strengthen muscles on each side of the lower abdomen.

Aiding Exercise with Water

Submerging your body in a pool of water will often make range of motion exercises easier. The buoyancy of the water will relieve pressure on joints and discs and reduce leverage on muscles and joints. Bending and twisting your trunk *slowly* while standing in chest-deep water can help relieve painful stiffness and swelling. The hydrostatic pressure of the water against your body will also aid circulation.

As you grow stronger and pain begins to subside, you can increase the resistance of water exercises by simply moving a little faster. When you can move about without pain, you may then gradually switch to resistive body weight exercises on land. From there, you can go on to a good progressive resistance barbell program if you are so inclined.

What to Do about Postural Kyphosis

A kyphosis is simply a slumped thoracic spine—or a hump back. If the slumping cannot be corrected with good posture (see Chapter 9), you should do a couple of special exercises with a barbell. For best results, do the exercises every other day or at least twice a week.

Slumping associated with structural changes in the spine cannot be fully corrected, but exercise and good posture can help prevent progressive deformity.

On the next page are four good barbell exercises that are designed to pull your upper spine into an erect position. You can make your own barbell by filling two gallon jugs with water or sand and placing them on each end of a broomstick. Control the amount of weight by adjusting the water level in each jug. For a maximum amount of weight, add water to sand-filled jugs.

1. Standing Press with a Barbell: Stand erect and press a barbell from shoulder level to overhead. Use enough weight to provide moderate resistance for eight to ten repetitions.

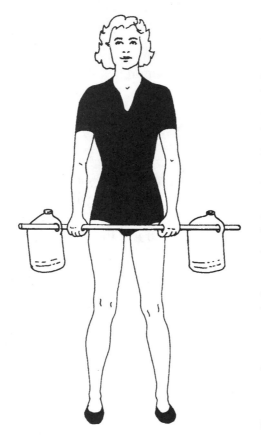

2. Shoulder Shrugs: Stand erect and hold a barbell down at arm's length in front. Shrug your shoulders up and down fifteen or twenty times. This exercise is especially effective for developing the muscles that support your shoulder girdle.

3. Upright Rowing Motions: Stand erect and hold a barbell down at arm's length in front. With a close, palms-down grip on the bar, lift the bar up to your neck, pointing your elbows up and out. Use only enough weight to permit eight to ten comfortable repetitions.

Upright rowing motions, along with standing presses with a barbell, will strengthen upper back muscles that help hold your spine erect.

Figure 7-5. Shrugging the shoulders up and down while holding a weight down at arm's length in front will strengthen supporting shoulder girdle muscles.

4. Straight-Arm Pullover: This exercise is similar to the exercise recommended in Chapter 4 for prevention of dowager's hump. Lie back over a thick cushion so that it supports you between your shoulder blades. Hold a light barbell (20 or 30 pounds) at arm's length over your chest. Holding your elbows in a slightly bent position, lower the weight back over your head to the floor while inhaling deeply. Return to starting position and repeat eight to ten times.

Resistive straight-arm pullovers will lift your chest and activate muscles that contribute greatly to improved posture.

What to Do about Swayback

Some swaybacks are structural in nature and cannot be corrected. Postural swayback, however, can often be corrected simply by standing tall and tucking the pelvis under a little.

Since both structural and postural swayback can place irritating pressure on spinal joints, such exercises as bent-knee sit-ups or bent-knee leg raises will often relieve discomfort by reversing the curve of the lower (lumbar) spine. Simply lying on your side and rolling up into a ball might provide some immediate relief from jamming of spinal joints.

Pelvic-tilting exercises, such as lying on your back with your knees bent and tilting your pelvis so that your lower back is pressed flat against the floor, might help relieve symptoms and retrain posture.

Try standing against a wall and tilting your pelvis so that your lower back is flattened against the wall.

Frog kicks, or hanging from a chinning bar and lifting your knees up toward your chest while curling your trunk will tilt your pelvis, reverse swayback, and stretch your spine to help correct postural imbalance.

Flexing your lumbar spine with hip-flexion exercises will relieve pressure on spinal joints, but excessive use of hip-flexion exercises might result in overdevelopment or shortening of hip-flexor muscles. This shortening might aggravate swayback by pulling the pelvis forward. So when you do hip-flexion exercises, you should always include some hip-extension exercises, such as those described in Chapter 5 and in this chapter.

Unless you are an athlete training to jump hurdles or perform some specialized skill, you really do not have to worry too much about developing a muscle imbalance when you do back exercises. But it's always a good idea to do a variety of exercises, including exercises that develop and stretch supporting muscles on each side of the spine.

Be sure to study the stretching exercises described in Chapter 5.

It Takes Time to Develop Back Muscles

Once you start an exercise program for your back, stick with it—provided, of course, that it does not cause pain or discomfort. Remember that it takes time to condition and strengthen muscles. It might take a couple of weeks to become accustomed to the exercises and then maybe another three or four weeks to see a measurable increase in strength.

Every-other-day exercise is usually best for building strength with an increase in muscle size. Frequency of training should never be less than twice a week.

It takes several weeks to condition a muscle but only a few weeks to lose conditioning. You may, in fact, begin to lose strength after only a week or two of inactivity. After several weeks, you may be back where you started. Obviously, an exercise program for your back should be a lifelong project. This is one reason I usually recommend only a few basic exercises that are easy and convenient to do. An overly enthusiastic or rigorous exercise program will soon be abandoned by most busy people.

Once the muscles supporting your spine have been strengthened by exercise, it does not take much exercise to maintain that strength. If you get a little tired of doing exercises on a regular basis, remember that if you just continue to do at least one basic exercise for each major muscle group, such as bent-knee sit-ups for your abdominal muscles, a hyperextension exercise for your back muscles, and simple squatting exercises for your thigh muscles, at least twice a week, you'll continue to have good muscle protection for your spine.

Keep Your Exercise Comfortable!

When an exercise causes pain, it's doing more harm than good. If you have a joint or facet problem in your spine, for example, hyperextension exercises might be painful. You may then have to substitute a back exercise that does not require back arching, such as facedown, one-legged, straight-leg lifts. If you have a bulging disc and forward bending causes back or leg pain, you may have to do trunk curls instead of sit-ups, and so on.

Protect Your Back in a Variety of Ways

While strong back muscles and correct lifting techniques will do a lot to protect your back from injury, remember that poor posture is a common cause of back pain. So is arthritis. Be sure to read the rest of this book if you want to do all you can to prevent or relieve backache.

SUMMARY

1. Muscles on all sides of the spine should be strengthened so that they support the spine in the same manner that guy wires support a radio tower.

2. The abdominal muscles are often the weakest of the muscles supporting the spine and may therefore require special attention.

3. Sit-up exercises should always be done with the knees *bent* in order to reduce the load on hip flexors and to reduce leverage on the lower back.

4. Bent-knee sit-ups, which use the hip flexors in a shortened position, should be followed by an exercise that *stretches* the hip flexors.

5. The spina erecta muscles on the back of your spine should have enough reserve strength to hold your spine erect and to perform daily tasks without becoming fatigued.

6. No matter how strong your back muscles might be, you should lift with your legs and not your back.

7. Squatting exercises to strengthen your leg muscles are just as important as back exercises to strengthen your spina erecta muscles in building protection for your lower back.

8. Overall body strength is necessary in order to protect your back and spine from awkward strains.

9. Basic barbell exercises provide a convenient and effective way to strengthen basic muscle groups while developing the muscles used in lifting.

10. Do not do any exercise that causes pain or that seems to place an awkward strain on your back.

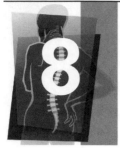

How to Handle
Spinal Arthritis in a
Self-Help Program

Arthritis is undoubtedly the most common of human ailments. With thirty-six million Americans suffering from arthritic symptoms, it appears that few of us will escape the pain and discomfort of inflamed joints as we grow older. With 150 joints connecting 206 bones in our skeletal structure, there is plenty of opportunity for arthritis or joint inflammation to develop. If we live long enough, we certainly won't be able to avoid arthritis caused by wear and tear on joint surfaces, especially in the 103 joints of the spine. Spinal arthritis is so common that we have a one-in-three chance of developing the disease by the age of thirty and a nine-in-ten chance by the age of seventy-five.

Common Forms of Spinal Arthritis

There are over one hundred types of arthritis, three of which commonly occur in the spine—osteoarthritis, rheumatoid arthritis, and ankylosing spondylitis. Osteoarthritis is an inflammation that results in the formation of bony spurs, while rheumatoid arthritis erodes joint cartilage. Ankylosing spondylitis causes the vertebrae to fuse or grow together.

When the symptoms of arthritis appear, they should be diagnosed medically, if not by your family physician, then by an orthopedic specialist or a rheumatologist. Such diseases as gout or systemic lupus erythematosus must be ruled out before a diagnosis of rheumatoid arthritis can be made.

Bone disease—and arthritis caused by infection—must also be considered. Soft tissue disorders such as cellulitis, myositis, fibrositis, and myofascitis also often cause symptoms similar to those seen in arthritis.

Wear-and-tear osteoarthritis, the most common and least serious form of spinal arthritis, can often be diagnosed by looking at plain spinal X rays.

To diagnose rheumatoid arthritis, your physician might order such blood studies as an erythrocyte sedimentation rate (ESR), a fluorescent anti-nuclear antibody (FANA) test, and a rheumatoid factor (RF) test.

Persons with lupus erythematosus might also have a positive FANA test along with a positive LE and a positive anti-DNA test.

The more serious condition of ankylosing spondylitis, which fuses the vertebrae together, might require a special serum HLA–B27 protein molecule gene test.

Obviously, your physician or a rheumatologist must order the appropriate tests to make the correct diagnosis—often through a process of elimination.

Fortunately, ankylosing spondylitis is less common than osteoarthritis and rheumatoid arthritis. Both ankylosing spondylitis and rheumatoid arthritis can be crippling and should be treated by a rheumatologist. Osteoarthritis, on the other hand, is rarely crippling and can be controlled with self-help.

If you are a young man and you begin to have morning back stiffness and back pain that is not relieved by lying down, and such symptoms persist longer than three months, ask your doctor for a blood arthritis profile to rule out ankylosing spondylitis. This disease is most common in young men.

When spinal arthritis of any type is acutely painful, anti-inflammatory drugs prescribed by a physician might be needed to allow the rest and the movement required to make life tolerable and to keep inflammation to a minimum.

Arthritis Treatment and Prevention at Home

In this chapter, you'll learn something about the three most common forms of spinal arthritis and what you can do about them.

Remember that most forms of arthritis cannot be cured. There are no magical remedies. There is plenty that you can do at home, however, to relieve symptoms and prevent disability. Good posture, correct lifting techniques, control of body weight, and other simple measures designed to avoid abnormal pressure or strain on your spine will help. Good nutrition provided by a low-fat, high-carbohydrate diet of fresh, natural foods that supply adequate vitamin C, calcium, and other nutrients needed for healthy joint cartilage and bone can make a big difference. Exercise to maintain joint mobility and to stimulate an increase in the strength of bone and cartilage can help prevent bony compression and crippling stiffness. (Too much exercise, however, can result in an increase in joint pain.)

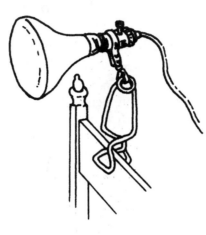

Figure 8-1. *A simple infrared heat lamp clamped to the back of a chair can be used to irradiate and heat a warm moist towel applied over any arthritic joint in the body.*

Moist heat applied to sore arthritic joints may alleviate much of the pain. When a moist heat application fails to relieve symptoms, a cold pack might do the job. Heat applications should be limited to twenty to thirty minutes; cold applications to ten to twenty minutes.

Except in the case of gouty arthritis, simple aspirin is believed to be the best and most effective medication for arthritis. Always try aspirin before resorting to more powerful anti-inflammatory drugs.

Like any drug, aspirin can have side effects. If you have a stomach ulcer or any other gastrointestinal problem, or if you are taking medication of any kind, you might be advised not to take aspirin. If you're taking a blood thinner, or if you have surgery pending, your doctor might substitute some other medication for aspirin—such as acetaminophen (Tylenol).

You should never take large doses of aspirin without your doctor's permission. Two aspirins every four hours are considered to be safe and effective for pain relief. Larger doses for anti-inflammatory effects should be prescribed by a physician. Depending upon the type and degree of arthritis you have, a physician who can monitor blood salicylate (aspirin) levels can prescribe the amount of aspirin that will be safe and effective for you.

A standard aspirin tablet is about 325 milligrams, or 5 grains, in size. An "arthritic strength" aspirin is simply a larger tablet, containing around 500 milligrams of aspirin instead of the usual 325 milligrams.

Aspirin should be taken with food to reduce chances of stomach irritation. If you have a stomach problem, a buffered or enteric-coated aspirin that does not dissolve until after it passes through the stomach might be best.

If you're not sure what type of spinal arthritis you have, be sure to read all of this chapter. Read a good book on arthritis written by a specialist who is associated with an accredited university or medical facility. Remember that there are many quacks offering a treatment for arthritis. Learn all you can about arthritis—and then see a specialist if necessary.

Most of what must be done to relieve the symptoms of arthritis must be done by *you*. Keep in mind that self-help in the care of arthritis is something you must do every day for the rest of your life.

Self-Help in the Care of Wear-and-Tear Osteoarthritis (OA)

Sid D., a sixty-one-year-old contractor, had been experiencing recurring backache for several years. Lately, however, he had been finding it difficult to rest comfortably in bed. When morning came, his spine was so stiff and painful that he literally had to roll out of bed. After a few hours on his feet, however, he felt fine—except for a little uncomfortable stiffness. Sitting for a few hours resulted in a return of painful stiffness, making it temporarily difficult for Sid to straighten up and move about. A little lifting or exertion on the job often resulted in muscle spasms in his lower back.

When Sid visited my office, he was in a panic. "My doctor says I have a degenerating spine," he wailed. "Am I going to end up in a wheelchair?"

Actually, Sid had degenerative osteoarthritis, which is just another name for Type M wear-and-tear arthritis, a degeneration of joint and disc cartilage that is accompanied by a buildup of bony ridges around the vertebrae. This type of arthritis is also often called spondylosis, degenerative disc disease (DDD), degenerative joint disease, osteoarthrosis, hypertrophic arthritis, old-age arthritis, or simply wear-and-tear arthritis. When inflammation is present, doctors might call the disease "osteoarthritis." When inflammation is *not* present, the disease might be called "osteoarthrosis."

I assured Sid that he could live with his arthritis and that he would not end up in a wheelchair. "If you have to have arthritis," I told Sid, "you have the best kind. We all get it sooner or later."

Diagnosing Spinal Osteoarthritis

Osteoarthritis shows up clearly on plain X-ray film but cannot be diagnosed with blood tests. Testing may be needed, however, to rule out rheumatoid arthritis or ankylosing spondylitis.

Although fearsome sounding in name, degenerative osteoarthritis is not as serious as other forms of spinal arthritis, since there is normally little inflammation and rarely fusion of joints. The disease may occur only in joints where stress is greatest, as in the lower portions of the neck and the lower back. Since disc herniation also occurs most often in these portions of the spine, your doctor must rule out collapse or prolapse of a disc before making a diagnosis of disc degeneration that is associated with degenerative osteoarthritis or spondylosis. The older you are, the more likely your problem is caused by degeneration rather than herniation of a disc.

Over sixteen million Americans suffer from osteoarthritis. More than half of the population will show signs of joint degeneration by the age of sixty. When arthritis involves the spinal joints, it's called degenerative joint disease (DJD), as opposed to degenerative disc disease (DDD). If a herniated disc is found on MRI (magnetic resonance imaging) or CAT (computerized axial tomography) studies, it might be called a herniated nucleus pulposus, or HNP. Ask your doctor for a copy of the medical report describing your back pain and see if you can figure out what it means.

Primary osteoarthritis is usually associated with aging and wear and tear and involves many joints. Most of us will experience this form of arthritis at some point in time.

Secondary osteoarthritis is more localized and usually occurs only in joints that have been sprained or injured. In the spine, joint deformities, curvatures, disc degeneration, and other conditions that overload spinal joints can result in secondary or localized osteoarthritis or arthrosis.

The Bony Overgrowth of Osteoarthritis

Once the symptoms of degenerative osteoarthritis begin to appear, usually after middle age, shrinking and aging intervertebral discs may begin to wear thin and degenerate, especially in the middle of the neck and the lower back. As a result, the vertebrae move closer together, narrowing the openings through which the spinal nerves pass. As the discs become thinner, joints begin to override each other and ligaments are placed under stress. Joint cartilage degenerates, allowing bone to rub against bone. As a result of this irritation, ridges of bone called osteophytes, or spurs, build up gradually around the vertebrae—much like a callus on your heel.

Fortunately, spurs are not often painful unless they are injured or disturbed. They will, however, sometimes encroach upon a spinal nerve to cause excruciating, radiating pain, usually down one arm or one leg. Severe bony ridging might also encroach upon the spinal canal, causing stenosis or narrowing of the canal. When bony overgrowth narrows an opening where a spinal nerve passes between two vertebrae, the condition might be called lateral spinal stenosis. When such narrowing occurs in the spinal canal (housing the spinal cord), it is called central spinal stenosis.

Thickening of ligaments (ligamentum flavum) on the back of the vertebrae can also encroach upon the spinal canal. So can Paget's disease, which causes an abnormal thickening of bone.

CAT scans have proven to be useful in detecting central spinal stenosis. If you're past middle age and you have weakness or cramping in both legs, ask your doctor to check you for neurogenic claudication, which is often caused by central spinal stenosis.

Watch for Nerve Root Involvement

Plain spinal X rays will readily show degenerative osteoarthritis and lateral spinal stenosis. When nerve root irritation is present, radiation of symptoms into an arm or a leg will clearly indicate a pinched nerve. Oblique X-ray views will often reveal the offending bony spur. (An MRI study is best for visualizing nerve root encroachment caused by a herniated disc.)

When symptoms radiate down both arms or both legs, or when there is weakness in the sphincter muscles that control the bladder or the bowels, a CAT or MRI scan might be needed to detect or rule out the presence of central spinal stenosis or the protrusion of a disc into the spinal canal.

Fortunately, central spinal stenosis is relatively rare, and the bony overgrowth of spinal osteoarthritis does not often cause serious problems. X-ray images often reveal severe degenerative changes in the spine of people who are not even aware of the problem. On the other hand, slight changes might be associated with severe pain or muscle spasm, depending upon the location of these changes. A small spur in a joint, or a spur projecting into a space occupied by a spinal nerve, for example, might cause big problems,

8

while a huge osteophyte (spur) on the body of a vertebra might be totally innocuous.

The changes that occur in degenerative osteoarthritis are, of course, permanent. A certain amount of chronic stiffness and aching is to be expected. But acute symptoms may come and go, depending upon the type of stress placed upon the spine. Even when a spinal nerve is pinched or irritated by a spur, the symptoms will often subside with time and rest. Formation of scar tissue might pad the crowded nerve, or symptoms might simply disappear when swelling subsides. When nerve pressure is not relieved in time, relief of pain might not occur until the involved nerve fibers die. A damaged spinal nerve can, of course, result in muscle weakness or sensory disturbance in the part of the body supplied by that particular nerve. Consultation with a neurologist or a neurosurgeon who can monitor nerve function can help you decide whether you should let time do the healing or submit to surgery to relieve symptoms and prevent nerve damage.

Common Home Treatments for Spinal Arthritis

Sid D. got along fine most of the time, despite some apparently severe arthritic changes in his spine. Whenever he experienced acute back pain after working in the yard or after a long trip, he usually recovered with rest and moist heat applications to his lower back.

Davy S. also suffered from degenerative osteoarthritis in the lower portion of his spine. Years of work as a longshoreman had literally worn out his lumbar discs. Large spurs projecting off his vertebrae were actually touching each other. Davy's back ached so badly most of the time that he was forced to take aspirin or Tylenol occasionally to relieve the pain. (Davy was aware that aspirin is an anti-inflammatory as well as a painkiller, while Tylenol is used primarily for pain relief.) He also wore a lumbar support when acute back pain made it difficult for him to move around. "I can't get by without my back support when I have a spell with my back," Davy admitted, "but I don't wear it all the time." He added, however, that he would occasionally wear the support when he had to work especially hard or be on his feet for a long period of time.

I instructed both Sid and Davy in the use of hot packs and cold packs. I told them how to lift properly and how to protect their spine with good posture.

"Simply switching to a good, firm mattress probably helped me more than anything," Sid reported.

Davy felt that a change in his sitting posture and the occasional use of a lumbar support kept him on his feet. "I know my back problem is something I have to live with," Davy admitted, "but I've learned that what I do to help myself can make the difference between being a cripple or being productive. In fact, my pain is not nearly as bad now as it was before I started observing the home treatment and prevention tips you gave me."

Just to make sure that Sid and Davy would continue to lead productive and pain-free lives, I gave them special exercises to strengthen their legs so that they could lift with their legs instead of with their back. (See Chapter 9 for correct lifting techniques.)

Practically everything you learn in every chapter of this book will help you in the treatment and prevention of wear-and-tear spinal arthritis. So be sure to read this entire book, even if you do not now have spinal arthritis and even if your doctor has told you that there is no cure for arthritis.

If you are overweight and you have spinal arthritis, it's essential that you reduce your body weight to relieve the load on your spinal joints (see Chapter 6).

Keep Moving to Preserve Flexibility

Remember that it's important to keep the joints of your spine moving, even when movement is a little painful. During the early stages of degenerative osteoarthritis, when the cartilage covering the joint surfaces is eroding or wearing away, the joints may be sore and stiff. After the cartilage has been worn away, the exposed bony surfaces may begin to harden, permitting more movement with less pain. So even if your spinal arthritis is acutely painful now, it might be less painful in the future. If you keep moving in order to stay as flexible as possible, you'll have better use of your spine when the pain finally subsides. Simple bending exercises may be all you need to do—preferably following moist heat applications or a hot shower.

An occasional gentle spinal manipulation might be beneficial in maintaining mobility in vertebral joints diseased by osteoarthritis. Such manipulation can be performed by a chiropractor, osteopath, physiatrist, or physical therapist.

Exercise is important in keeping bones strong as well as to maintain mobility. The inactivity induced by painful spinal arthritis drains calcium from the vertebrae. Make sure that you have plenty of calcium in your diet. (Taking calcium supplements will not increase the size and formation of arthritic spurs.) When dietary calcium is deficient, calcium will be pulled from your bones to form the bony spurs of arthritis, thus weakening your bones with osteoporosis.

How to Cope with Inflammatory Rheumatoid Arthritis (RA)

Shelia B., a thirty-year-old housewife, had been diagnosed as having spinal rheumatoid arthritis. While her X rays did not look as bad as those of someone suffering from degenerative osteoarthritis, her form of arthritis was more serious and more crippling.

In rheumatoid arthritis, there are no bony spurs or overgrowths. Instead, in the beginning, there is a barely perceptible erosion of joints with much inflammation and swelling in the synovial membranes surrounding the joints. This inflammation literally destroys the joint cartilage, discs, and supporting tissues, resulting in crippling, painful stiffness with deformity.

The cause of rheumatoid arthritis is unknown, but it may have a systemic or viral origin, triggering an autoimmune reaction—a Type O arthritis. This is why victims of rheumatoid arthritis often feel tired, sick, and feverish. Shelia B., for example, complained of backache and neckache that was accompanied by fever and other symptoms of illness. Her family physician, a first-class medical sleuth, ordered a special rheumatoid factor test after ruling out infection, thus establishing the diagnosis.

Age and Sex a Factor in Rheumatoid Arthritis

The symptoms of rheumatoid arthritis usually appear between the ages of thirty and fifty. It occurs in about 1 percent of the population, most often in women. Whenever a young woman or a young man complains of persistent backache or neckache of unknown origin, I usually order tests for rheumatoid arthritis. The joints of the fingers, hands, wrists, elbows, shoulders, knees, ankles, and feet are most commonly affected by rheumatoid arthritis. The disease also develops in the neck.

Once diagnosed, a person with rheumatoid arthritis should be placed under the care of a rheumatologist, a medical doctor who specializes in the diagnosis and treatment of arthritis and other diseases that inflame muscles and joints. There is no known cure for rheumatoid arthritis, which is usually a lifelong disease, but special medication to reduce inflammation may be helpful in reducing destruction and relieving pain. Sometimes, the disease will go into complete remission, with or without treatment.

Nonsteroidal anti-inflammatory drugs such as aspirin or ibuprofen are commonly prescribed. When aspirin does not work or is not appropriate, your doctor might prescribe more powerful anti-inflammatory drugs, such as steroids or corticosteroids.

Cold packs applied over painful joints will sometimes relieve pain by reducing inflammation or by numbing nerves. In less acute cases, moist heat might be more effective. Special exercises following the application of heat or cold might be needed to keep the diseased joints mobile.

Beware of Neck Manipulation

Gentle manipulation of the spine might be helpful when symptoms are not acute, but neck manipulation should be avoided. When the joints of the neck or cervical spine are infected by active rheumatoid arthritis, inflammation in the membranes surrounding the joints might weaken supporting ligaments and dissolve joint cartilage. The result is that the atlas, the upper most vertebra supporting the skull, might actually become loose and displaced, endangering the spinal cord. Manipulation of the neck could result in dislocation of the atlas, causing death or paralysis.

If you have a painful neck and you have rheumatoid arthritis, see an orthopedic specialist for neck X rays in case your neck is becoming dangerously unstable.

How Shelia B. Helped Herself in the Treatment of Her Arthritis

Shelia was placed under the care of a rheumatologist, but she did a lot at home to help herself. When her neck and back pains were mild, she used moist heat (twenty to thirty minutes) over her spine. When pain was acute, she applied cold packs (fifteen to twenty minutes) to reduce inflammation and numb the pain. She used aspirin to relieve pain and combat inflammation.

"My rheumatologist told me not to take strong painkillers," Shelia explained. "He told me that pain helps protect the joints by discouraging overuse. So I expect to have a certain amount of pain. I use pain as a guide in deciding how much exercise to do."

Remember, however, that when rheumatoid arthritis is severe, it might be necessary to take prescription anti-inflammatory medication to reduce joint destruction.

Maintain Mobility with Special Exercises

Shelia had learned an important lesson in caring for her arthritis. She knew that a certain amount of exercise is needed to keep the joints from developing permanent adhesions. She also knew that rest is needed to reduce inflammation. Too much rest, however, weakens muscles and bones and makes exercise more difficult. So Shelia avoided the use of painkillers, and she exercised as much as she could without triggering a painful reaction. Arthritis specialists generally agree that *if exercise causes pain that lasts longer than two hours, you have either done too much exercise or the wrong kind of exercise.*

The best exercise program is one that can be done at home. Such exercise should always be regulated according to the amount of pain or discomfort you experience.

The inflammation of rheumatoid arthritis tends to subside or disappear with time—after a few months or years. It's important, however, to exercise your muscles and joints to prevent permanent stiffness before the disease "burns out."

Shelia's Simple Exercise Program

Shelia had a very simple but effective exercise program. Each day she moved her spine in every direction. She rotated her head to the right and to the left several times and then bent her neck forward and backward a few times. To move the rest of her spine, she would lean forward and touch her shins and then lean backward a little. She would also bend from side to side and then twist to one side and then to the other. Shelia did her exercises slowly and deliberately, being careful to keep the exercise comfortable and to avoid excessive momentum.

It's always best to do simple exercises that duplicate normal, everyday movements. Don't roll your head around, touch your toes, or attempt to do an awkward or difficult exercise. Any exercise you do should be designed to move your joints through a normal range of movement and to maintain muscle tone rather than stretch tendons or build muscles. Keep your exercise gentle, comfortable, and practical.

Using a Special Neck Pillow

Because rheumatoid arthritis had spread into her neck, Shelia searched until she found a comfortable pillow that would evenly support the back of her head and her neck. She made sure that her neck remained in line with the rest of her spine, whether she was lying on her back or on her side. Sleeping face down was out of the question, since this position placed too much strain on her neck.

See Chapter 3 for more information on neck pillows and neck care.

When Symptoms Go into Remission

As the years went by, Shelia's neck pain subsided, and she seemed to recover with only a small amount of stiffness. Remember, however, that the course of rheumatoid arthritis is unpredictable. Symptoms may subside and recur for no apparent reason, with or without treatment. So don't jump to the conclusion that you have been cured by a home remedy when symptoms subside temporarily. Persons who claim that an unorthodox remedy has cured their arthritis might simply be experiencing a remission of symptoms.

It's well known that the symptoms of rheumatoid arthritis will often subside or surge according to the amount of stress experienced. If you are a victim of rheumatoid arthritis, try to maintain a happy, carefree attitude. Keep stress to a minimum, but resolve to deal with stress firmly and confidently so that you are always in control. There is some evidence to indicate that uncontrolled stress, causing anxiety, loss of sleep, panic, or a reduction in self-esteem, can trigger a systemic reaction that can activate rheumatoid arthritis.

We cannot avoid stress, but we can avoid letting it whip us into a sick, defensive state.

The Bamboo Spine of Ankylosing Spondylitis (AS)

Ankylosing spondylitis is less common than osteoarthritis and rheumatoid arthritis and occurs twice as often in men as in women. Unlike rheumatoid arthritis, which may begin in the neck and upper back, *ankylosing spondylitis almost always begins in the sacroiliac joints at the bottom of the spine.* From there, the disease gradually works its way up the spine, sometimes involving only a few vertebrae and sometimes spreading all the way to the neck.

As ankylosing spondylitis progresses, the inflamed vertebrae may fuse together, leaving the spine solid and stiff. When the entire spine is affected, the victim is unable to stand erect and must turn his entire body to turn his head.

8

Also known as Marie-Strumpell disease or poker spine, this terrible disease usually begins at a young age, most often in men in their twenties or thirties, affecting less than 1 percent of the population. The cause of this Type O disease is unknown and it may be inherited. There is no known cure. Early detection of the disease, however, will help prevent deformity by allowing prompt, proper treatment with postural exercises and anti-inflammatory drugs.

Diagnosing Ankylosing Spondylitis

Timothy T. was only twenty-two years of age when he began to complain of low-back aching. Regular medical checkups did not reveal a cause for his back trouble. After a few years of gradually increasing back pain, Timothy finally visited an orthopedic specialist who ordered a special blood test. "Persons suffering from ankylosing spondylitis have an HLA–B27 protein molecule gene in their blood," the specialist explained. "If you have rheumatoid arthritis, you'll have a rheumatoid factor in your blood, but you won't have the B27 gene."

Such tests are important in distinguishing between rheumatoid arthritis and ankylosying spondylitis, since changes in X-ray readings may not appear early in either disease. In the case of ankylosing spondylitis, the sacroiliac joints (just below your last vertebra) will eventually begin to show signs of inflammation and fusion.

There is a simple physical test that is often helpful in diagnosing ankylosing spondylitis. Since this disease tends to fuse rib cartilage together, chest expansion is reduced. When *chest expansion is less than two inches* (from inhaling to exhaling), tests for ankylosing spondylitis might be ordered.

For some unknown reason, eye inflammation often accompanies ankylosing spondylitis.

As the disease becomes more advanced, X-ray changes become more apparent. If the disease spreads from the sacroiliac joints, the discs between the vertebrae are destroyed and replaced by fibrous tissue that gradually turns to bone, fusing the vertebrae together. Bulging of the bony discs and ligaments makes the X-ray image of the spine look as if were a stalk of bamboo, thus the expression "bamboo spine."

Keeping the Spine Straight

Sometimes ankylosing spondylitis will spread only part way up the spine, causing only partial stiffness. Too often, however, the disease fuses the entire spine into a solid mass, making it impossible to bend or look around. Obviously, good posture and special exercises are very important in the early stages of the disease if erect posture is to be preserved. Deep breathing exercises may be needed to keep the rib cage flexible. It's absolutely essential that a victim of ankylosing spondylitis sit, stand, and sleep in postures that keep the spine as straight as possible, otherwise a permanent stooped posture may develop. Special medication might be needed to reduce the pain that discourages an erect posture. This is one reason it's so important to be under the care of a rheumatologist who can prescribe non-steriodal anti-inflammatory medication (such Indocin) as well as exercise.

How Timothy T. Prevented Spinal Deformity Through Early Diagnosis and Self-help Measures

Timothy was fortunate in having his ankylosing spondylitis diagnosed early enough to get proper treatment. Although the progress of the disease was not altered by the treatment, Timothy was able to avoid serious spinal deformity. "I kept my spine as straight as possible at all times," he explained. "I never stayed bent over for very long. When I went to bed at night, I slept flat on my back on a firm bed so that I could keep my spine in alignment. I took deep breathing exercises every day, and I stretched my chest muscles by throwing my shoulders back. I also did bending exercises every day after a hot bath, moving my spinal joints through a full range of movement in every direction. Although my spine is partially stiff, I'm standing fairly straight."

Luckily for Timothy, his spondylitis burned out about half way up his spine. He was spared the total fusion that freezes the neck along with the rest of the spine.

Good posture and exercise are probably the two most important measures you can take to keep your spine from freezing in a tilted posture. Since the disease may smolder or progress for ten to twenty years before burning out, it's important to make good posture and corrective exercise a part of your way of life. If you're lucky, the disease may burn out before it transverses your entire spine.

The straight-arm pullover exercise described in Chapter 7 might be helpful in expanding your rib cage and keeping your thoracic spine straight.

Remember that while exercise is important, it's also important to avoid exhaustion. Make sure that you get adequate rest each day—both mentally and physically. Make a special effort to avoid staying in postures in which your spine is slumped and your head is down. Be sure to avoid sleeping on a thick pillow with your neck flexed (your chin on your chest).

Gouty Arthritis and Backache

We normally think of gout as a disease affecting only the big toe, the wrist, the knee, or some other joint in an arm or a leg.

Gout can, however, cause or aggravate back pain. When spinal gouty arthritis does occur, the pain that results can be severe. X rays may be negative and there may be no physical or musculoskeletal clue pointing to the cause of the pain.

Diagnosing and Controlling Gout

Actually, gout is a systemic or metabolic disease, requiring a blood test for diagnosis. Medication might also be needed for relief of pain. Since the development of gout signals the onset of a failure in the body's ability to metabolize and eliminate uric acid, there is no cure for the disease, which must be kept under control by diet or by drugs.

Normally, uric acid in the blood does not rise above a certain level, the excess being excreted by the kidneys. When body metabolism produces an excessive amount of uric acid, or when the kidneys fail to eliminate uric acid, the blood level rises so high that uric acid crystals accumulate in the tissues. When some of these crystals get into the joints, sudden severe pain may develop.

When gout involves a joint in an extremity, the skin around the swollen joint may be tight, shiny, and bright red or purple. And the involved joint may be so painful that the touch of bed sheets cannot be tolerated. The effect is much like that of having sand or ground glass between sensitive joint surfaces.

A uric acid test will usually reveal a level higher than seven milligrams per 100 milliliters of blood serum. Colchicine is often prescribed during the first two days of an attack of gouty arthritis—often with dramatic results in relief of pain. In chronic and severe cases of gout in which the body produces too much uric acid, allopurinol might be prescribed to block production of uric acid.

Nonsteroidal anti-inflammatory drugs, such as Indocin, might be substituted for colchicine. Aspirin is not recommended as a treatment for gout, since it tends to block urinary excretion of uric acid.

The Role of Diet in Gout

Although uric acid can be formed from the purines supplied by protein foods, especially meats, the foods you eat are not the primary cause of gout. Simply eating large amounts of meat will not cause gout in a healthy person. But once a person develops gout because of a metabolic disorder, eating large amounts of any purine-rich food can trigger an attack of gout. It may then be necessary to drastically reduce your intake of such foods as beans, lentils, fish, fowl, sardines, liver, gravies, and sweetbreads (animal pancreas or thymus).

While the metabolic defect that causes gout cannot be corrected, keeping your intake of meats to a minimum may reduce the frequency and the severity of the attacks, thus reducing your need for medication. Some gout victims might prefer to take medication regularly to keep serum uric acid under control so that they can continue to eat as they wish. Such drugs can have side effects, however, so it's always best to first try controlling gout with diet. A good low-fat, high-carbohydrate diet with no more than 12 to 15 percent of your intake coming from protein foods (see Chapter 6) will help prevent overweight, heart disease, cancer, and stroke, as well as gout.

If you suspect that you might have gouty arthritis, you should reduce your intake of meat and other foods derived from meat. You can get most of the protein you need from skim milk, eggs, and low-fat cheese, along with combinations of fruits, vegetables, and whole-grain products.

Drink lots of water every day to help your kidneys flush out excess uric acid—and to help prevent uric acid kidney stones as well as gout.

Body Weight and Gout

If you're overweight, remember that rapid loss of body weight can raise the level of uric acid in your blood. So don't go on a crash diet if you have gout. Even if you do not now have any of the symptoms of gout, keep weight loss down to a couple of pounds a week to avoid the release of too much uric acid (which is caused by the burning of protein and fat cells).

Most gouty arthritis occurs in men middle-aged and older who naturally tend to have a higher level of serum uric acid. Only about 5 percent of gout victims are women, most of whom have been through menopause. (One of the worst cases of gout I have ever seen occurred in a menopausal woman whose favorite dish was chili and beans, which is high in purines.)

When the symptoms of gout first develop, the first few attacks may last only a few days, disappearing without any special treatment. But as the disease becomes more advanced, attacks may become more painful and more frequent. If you have recurring back pain with no known cause, ask your doctor to check you for gouty arthritis, especially if you have a history of gout.

Myofascitis and Other Muscle Problems

The symptoms of fibromyositis, myositis, myofascitis, and other muscle conditions are often associated with or mistaken for arthritis. Postural strain, emotional stress, cold drafts, systemic disorders, and other factors can play a role in the development of muscle inflammation. Often, the causes of muscular complaints are not known. In recent years, the most popular label for chronic muscle inflammation has been "myofascitis," which doctors believe is commonly caused by unrelieved stress or tension. It's well known that prolonged, unrelieved muscle tension causes fatigue that inflames muscles with lactic acid.

Fibromyalgia is currently a popular diagnosis. This disease is characterized by fatigue, depression, and generalized muscle and joint pain, often a cause of chronic low-back pain. There is no medical test for fibromyalgia and no real cure. Many of the home remedies described in this book, such as exercise and moist heat, may relieve symptoms, but in extreme cases it may be necessary to seek prescription medication.

For an explanation of how the mind can influence the symptoms of fibromyalgia, see The Mind/Body Connection sidebar on page 255.

Polymyositis, a relatively rare generalized inflammation of muscles that causes fatigue and weakness, can involve the muscles of the neck and upper back. This condition is a systemic disease, like rheumatoid arthritis or lupus, and should be treated by a physician. The cause is unknown, but may be an immune system problem.

Polymyalgia rheumatica, a sudden onset of constant aching in the muscles of the neck, shoulders, hips, lower back, and buttocks that occurs for no apparent reason in persons over age fifty, is often self-limiting, but may last for years. When fever and other symptoms are present, a physician should be consulted for a definite diagnosis. This disease is often associated with temporal arteritis, a cause of head pain and a potentially serious problem (see Chapter 2).

Exercises, moist heat, massage, good posture, and freedom from emotional stress are all important in the treatment of chronic muscle tension.

There is now some evidence to indicate that when you laugh tension is relieved and muscles relax. Happy people who laugh a lot are less subject to rheumatoid arthritis and chronic muscle inflammation. Try to make happiness a part of your treatment program. Plan your activities so that you can do some of the things you like to do. Think positive, be optimistic, and concentrate on enjoying the gift of life.

Coping with Varieties of Muscle Inflammation

Symptoms of muscle inflammation in the shoulder blade area are often called fibrositis, fibromyositis, or myositis. Muscle spasm caused by inflamed muscles in the neck is sometimes called torticollis, which is the same as the "crick" discussed in Chapter 3. Muscle inflammation in the low-back area might be called "lumbago." Be sure to read Chapters 2 and 3 if your neck muscles are painful, and Chapter 4 if you have a backache.

Fibrositis or myofascitis most commonly occurs around the neck and shoulders, and it's often caused by postural strain or by emotional stress. People who work in prolonged static postures, for example, often develop inflamed muscles from unrelieved muscle tension. The most severe cases of myofascitis I have seen, however, have been caused by emotional stress.

How Molly D. Eased Her Neck Pain by Addressing Emotional Stress

Molly D. has been hospitalized twice for severe muscle spasm in her neck and upper back. X rays and other tests were negative, but the pain persisted. Injections into "trigger points" provided only temporary relief. Sometimes the pain and spasm would disappear, only to return a few days later. It soon became apparent that Molly's neck pain was caused by emotional stress. An unfaithful husband and a daughter on drugs kept Molly in constant mental agony. Difficulty sleeping and inability to relax during the day created muscle tightness that soon triggered painful spasms.

When Molly realized that her mental state was causing her physical problems, she was better able to handle both problems. "Now that I'm making a special effort to cope with my personal problems," she explained, "my therapy seems to be more effective. I'm using moist heat and taking regular exercise for my shoulder and neck muscles and I'm getting better! I know that when I get my head on straight, my pain will probably disappear. At least I know what's causing the pain, and I'm no longer inclined to run to the hospital emergency room every time I have a muscle spasm."

Sleeping with Arthritis

Spinal arthritis often interferes with sleep. Lying in one position for very long soon begins to cause discomfort or pain, making it necessary to change positions frequently. It's rarely necessary to take painkillers, sleeping pills, or sedatives to encourage sleep. When you get tired enough, you'll sleep. You'll also find that you can get by with less sleep than you thought. Besides, taking pain pills to deaden your nerves might only increase irritation in inflamed spinal joints by allowing you to stay in one position too long. It's good to move about and change positions frequently when your joints begin to ache.

A Firm Mattress, Sex, and Other Remedies

You should always make sure that you have a good, moderately firm mattress to sleep on. If you have a mate, twin beds might be a good idea to assure uninterrupted rest. Remember that your bed should be firm enough to keep your spine from sagging but not so hard that it cannot mold itself to the contours of your body. A bed that's too hard might allow your spine to sag in its unsupported portions.

A warm bath and a glass of wine at bedtime might help promote relaxation. According to recent news releases, a little alcohol might also help prevent heart disease—if overindulgence is avoided. You should not use alcohol of any kind if you cannot limit yourself to one or two drinks a day.

Sexual activities have proven to be beneficial for some victims of arthritis. "Sex loosens my spine," claims Sid D. "I'm convinced that sex is good therapy for arthritis. Besides, it makes a great line for a fellow my age!"

Some doctors believe that in addition to the exercise provided by sexual activity, a sexual orgasm relieves pain and reduces inflammation by triggering the release of certain hormones. Unlike the use of alcohol, it may be difficult or impossible to overindulge in sex. Chapter 11 deals with sex and back pain.

When pain is severe and you are taking aspirin as an anti-inflammatory drug, you can take two aspirin with a light meal at bedtime. Make sure, however, that your aspirin is pure and is not combined with caffeine or some ingredient that might interfere with sleep. When aspirin cannot be taken with a meal, chances of stomach irritation can be reduced by dissolving the aspirin in a glass of milk or juice.

There is some evidence to indicate that the amino acid tryptophane, supplied by milk, might help induce sleep.

Don't drink coffee, tea, colas, or cocoa in the evening, lest you be kept awake by caffeine. You need all the sleep you can get in order to reduce nervous irritability that might intensify your pain.

Systemic Lupus Erythematosus (SLE): The Great Pretender

Most of us don't think about lupus when we have chronic backache. But if you have undiagnosed backache, neck pain, or muscle or joint pain with occassional fever and other generalized symptoms, your doctor might order special blood tests to rule out systemic lupus. It's not unusual for patients to spend years undergoing treatment for arthritis and other diagnoses only to discover that they have systemic lupus, a disease that mimics the symptoms of many other diseases—organic and mechanical.

In addition to affecting muscles and joints, lupus can affect the collagen or connective tissue in the skin, kidneys, heart, lungs, nervous system, and other organs. The cause of lupus is unknown, although it is known to be an autoimmune disease in which the body's immune system attacks its own tissues. Since its symptoms are so varied, doctors sometimes call lupus "the great pretender." It is primarily a disease of young women.

If you have joint pains, flulike aching, hair loss (alopecia), headaches with skin rashes, and other nonspecific aches and pains that defy diagnosis, it might be a good idea to undergo antinuclear antibody testing for lupus.

A skin rash across the bridge of the nose and cheeks in a butterfly pattern is a characteristic lupus symptom.

When lupus is limited to skin involvement, it is called discoid lupus; when it involves joints and organs, it's called systemic lupus erythematosus.

Although there is no cure for lupus, there are treatments for the joint inflammation and other symptoms of the disease. It's essential that the correct diagnosis be made to facilitate treatment for possible organ involvement and to make sure that the disease is not mistaken for some other disease, such as rheumatoid arthritis.

SUMMARY

1. There are over one hundred types of arthritis, but osteoarthritis, rheumatoid arthritis, and ankylosing spondylitis are the most common forms of spinal arthritis.

2. With time and age, almost everyone will develop some degree of wear-and-tear spinal osteoarthritis.

3. In spinal osteoarthritis, the disc cartilage degenerates and the vertebrae build up ridges of bone, but these changes do not always cause problems.

4. In rheumatoid arthritis, inflammation in the synovial membranes surrounding the joints produces chemicals that erode cartilage and bone.

5. Ankylosing spondylitis, which is fairly rare, is an inflammatory process that begins in the sacroiliac joints and works its way up the spine, fusing joints as it goes along.

6. Although there is no cure for arthritis, there is plenty that you can do at home to relieve symptoms and maintain mobility.

7. Moist heat is generally best for relieving the soreness and stiffness of spinal arthritis and muscle spasm, but in cases of acute inflammation where there is throbbing pain, a cold pack might be more effective in relieving pain.

8. It's important to protect an arthritic spine from strain by avoiding excessive fatigue, bad posture, and heavy exertion.

9. Special exercises are important in maintaining mobility in diseased spinal joints, but it's important to balance rest and exercise so that exercise does not do more harm than good.

10. It's okay to take two aspirin occasionally to relieve pain, but you need a physician's guidance to take large doses of aspirin as an anti-inflammatory agent.

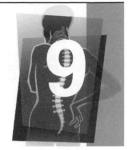

How to Prevent Back Strain by Using Proper Sitting, Standing, Lifting, and Sleeping Postures

Good posture is essential in the treatment and prevention of back trouble, whether you're sitting, standing, lifting, or lying down. The four curves in your spine, while balancing your vertebrae in an incredibly flexible and efficient structure, may actually increase susceptibility to injury when placed in improper positions. Consequently, you must be ever alert to avoid positions that place awkward or excessive strains on your back and spine.

As intelligent creatures with diverse capabilities, the conscious effort we make to protect our spine is well worth the gift of upright posture and the use of our hands. No other animal has a spine like a human. Even the gorilla, who can assume an upright posture, has only one curve in his spine.

While a single curve probably makes life less complicated and back trouble less likely for a gorilla, none of us would exchange our delicately balanced spinal curves and our erect posture for a primitive but stronger backbone. Besides, just imagine what the human shape would be like without spinal curves. In addition to increasing flexibility and mobility in an upright posture, the curves of the spine add to the shape and the beauty of the body—except when they are exaggerated by bad posture.

9

Protect Your Spinal Curves with Good Posture

In order to maintain the beauty of your body and the integrity of your spine with as little back trouble as possible, it's absolutely essential that you pay close attention to your posture. The curves that give your spine its special qualities can also be a source of pain when posture is bad. A slumped posture, for example, while appropriate for a gorilla with one spinal curve, will place a strain on your spine. Lying on a saggy mattress will strain joints and ligaments in certain portions of your spine. The same flexibility that allows you to bend in every direction can result in a back injury when you lift improperly. Even sitting must be carefully controlled to avoid damaging pressure or strain on muscles, joints, ligaments, and discs.

Because of the delicate balance in a flexible, curved spine, *bad posture and improper lifting techniques are two of the most common causes of backache and back strain.* No matter how strong your muscles are, you're going to have some back trouble if you do not use your spine properly.

In this chapter, I'll tell you how to protect your back from injury by doing nothing more than assuming a correct posture when you sit, stand, walk, lie down, or lift an object. Many cases of chronic or severe backache have resulted from such simple things as sitting in a bad chair, lying on a soft bed, or bending over to lift something. With proper attention to all these factors, you'll improve your physical appearance as well as prevent back trouble.

How Candace, Zack, and Allen Relieved Back Pain Caused by Poor Posture

Candace R. had chronic backache that was caused by sitting and watching television hour after hour in a poorly designed reclining chair. A little arthritis in her spine was being aggravated by a slumped posture. Since Candace wouldn't give up her TV shows, a new chair that supported the curve of her lower back solved her problem and relieved her pain.

After unsuccessful treatment by a number of doctors, Zack T. got rid of his chronic back problem by buying a new, firm mattress and changing his sleeping posture.

Allen R. normally got along fine with his back—except when he would lean over and reach out to lift something with his arms. Once, when he reached into the trunk of his car to lift out a sack of groceries, he suffered a back injury that kept him off the job for two weeks. It turned out that Allen had a structural abnormality in his lower spine, resulting in an instability that could not withstand the leverage of improper lifting.

Candace, Zack, and Allen were able to relieve and prevent their aches and pains simply by making a few postural changes—something anyone can do!

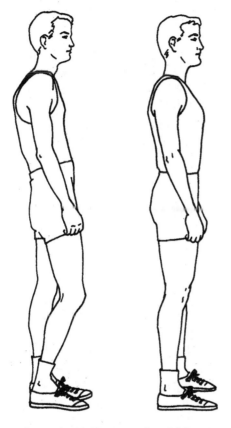

Figure 9-1. *Bad posture, in addition to causing chronic back pain, can detract from physical appearance and reflect lack of self-confidence.*

If you have spinal arthritis or any of the other spinal problems discussed in other chapters of this book, proper posture will be especially important in your back-care program. Such simple self-help measures as sitting properly and lifting correctly can often make the difference between being free from pain or spending hundreds of dollars seeking relief in doctors' offices. So be sure to study this chapter carefully. Don't discount something as simple and fundamental as posture improvement in the treatment and prevention of your back pain.

A Simple Rule for Maintaining Good Standing Posture

The four curves of the spine are normally evident in good posture. When the spine is viewed from the side, there is a cervical concavity on the back of the neck, a thoracic convexity between the shoulder blades, a lumbar concavity in the lower back, and a sacral convexity behind the pelvis. With good posture, these curves are minimal. But when posture slumps, all of these curves may be greatly exaggerated, resulting in what doctors refer to as cervical hyperlordosis, thoracic kyphosis, lumbar hyperlordosis, and sacral prominence.

As you know from reading other chapters of this book, there should not be any spinal curves from side to side, that is, when the spine is viewed from the back. When such curves are present, they may be the result of a scoliosis, a leg deficiency, or a muscle spasm caused by a back problem.

The normal curves of the spine may, of course, be more pronounced in some persons than in others and still be normal for the individual. So you should not expect postural curves to be exactly the same in everyone.

It would be a mistake to make a forced voluntary effort to flatten the curves in your spine. Pulling your chin in or your shoulders back, for example, or flattening your back against a wall, usually produces an abnormal posture that cannot be maintained voluntarily for very long.

In order to make the best use of your posture and the curves that are normal for you, *it's enough to simply stand tall in maintaining good posture.* A conscious effort to be as tall as you can be, without slumping, will hold you erect without distorting your normal curves.

Support Good Posture with Strong Muscles and Good Habits

Although good posture should not require much conscious muscular effort, you should have strong, well-developed muscles if you want to avoid end-of-the-day fatigue that causes you to slump from exhaustion. Any of the exercises described in other chapters of this book, such as the straight-arm pullover (Chapter 4), the shoulder shrug (Chapter 7), the prone hyperextension exercise (Chapter 7), and so on, will contribute to the development and maintenance of good posture.

For the most part, good posture is maintained by habit. In other words, you must consciously practice standing tall until you can do so without thinking about your posture. If you tend to have relaxed abdominal muscles or a prominent abdomen, you may also have to develop the habit of holding your abdomen in slightly. No matter how good your physical condition might be, your abdomen will tend to protrude when your abdominal muscles are totally relaxed. So even if you have well-developed abdominal muscles, try to cultivate the habit of holding your abdomen in just enough to keep your abdomen flat.

If your abdominal muscles are weak and flabby from lack of exercise, you'll have a potbelly even if you're not fat. This is one reason sit-up exercises are such an important part of a postural exercise program. You already know from reading Chapter 6 that carrying the off-center weight of a potbelly places a strain on your lower back, no matter how straight you stand or how strong your muscles are. (Ten pounds of potbelly, 10 inches away from the spine, places a 50-pound pull on the muscles on the back of the spine! This is a good example of how a slight imbalance in postural weight can strain muscles and joints.)

A potbelly caused by weak abdominal muscles can be corrected with exercise and muscle control. But if you want to get rid of a potbelly caused by a buildup of body fat, you may have to change your eating habits as well as exercise regularly.

Help Your Posture by Helping Your Feet

Believe it or not, the condition of your feet can have a lot to do with the type of posture you have. If you have weak ankles or fallen arches, for example, a rolling in of your ankles tends to rotate your legs inward, bringing your knees together and tilting your pelvis forward. This causes a lumbar swayback that results in compensatory exaggeration of your thoracic and cervical curves. A chain reaction then contributes to the development of aches and pains from your feet to your head. Tension headache is commonly associated with poor posture that places tension on the muscles of the neck. Obviously, you cannot afford to neglect your feet if you want truly good, pain-free posture.

You can keep your feet strong with regular heel-raising exercises—that is, by rising up and down on your toes. Go barefoot as much as possible. If you have weak or fallen arches, wear arch supports in your shoes. In many cases, the ready-made arch supports sold in drugstores will provide adequate support.

Try to point your toes fairly straight ahead when you walk. Make sure that your shoes conform to the shape of your foot, with adequate space for your toes.

Ladies should remember that wearing high-heeled shoes tends to cause swayback by tilting the pelvis forward. Medium or low heels are best.

If you have been wearing high-heeled shoes for many years, you may not be able to suddenly switch to low heels. When ankle tendons have been shortened by years of wearing high heels, lowering the heels all of a sudden might cause backache by transmitting a pull from the ankles to the lower back. Don't switch from high heels to low heels without first spending a few weeks doing the ankle-stretching exercises described in Chapter 5.

It might also be a good idea to stretch your hamstrings. I do not recommend toe-touching exercises, however, since forced flexion places compression on lumbar discs. When you bend forward, the first 60 degrees or so of flexion takes place in the lumbar spine, with an additional 20 degrees in the hip joints. If your hamstrings are tight or too short, flexion at the hips will be greatly restricted, preventing more than 60 degrees of forward bending. Any effort to force further bending will increase lumbar flexion, greatly increasing pressure on lumbar discs.

You can stretch your hamstrings safely and without placing compression on your lumbar discs by doing a "good morning exercise." You simply bend forward with your head up, your hands on your hips, and your legs locked out straight while maintaining an arch in your lower back. All the bending takes place in the hips, with none in the lower back. Lean forward until you feel a stretch in the muscles on the back of your legs.

How to Tilt Your Pelvis to Relieve Backache

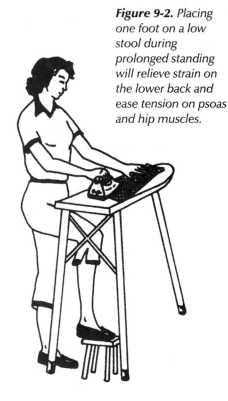

Figure 9-2. *Placing one foot on a low stool during prolonged standing will relieve strain on the lower back and ease tension on psoas and hip muscles.*

Standing in one position for a long time tends to cause backache by tilting the pelvis forward. Simply placing one foot up on a chair rung or on a low stool or a box will help prevent such backache by tilting the pelvis backward a little. Bending one knee might also relieve tension on a sensitive sciatic nerve. This is one reason bar foot rails were once installed in saloons—to permit drinkers to stand relaxed and pain free hour after hour at the bar.

If you have a job where you must stand for hours at a time, place a low stool or a wooden box at your feet so that you can reverse the tilt of your pelvis occasionally by resting one foot higher than the other.

How Edwin D. Relieved His Backache by Using a Footstool

Edwin D., a machinist who spent several hours a day standing at a drill press, relieved his backache by placing a footstool near his machine. "When my back begins to hurt, I get instant relief by placing one of my feet up on the stool," he proclaimed. "I got the idea from an orthopedic surgeon who uses such a stool when he performs lengthy surgery."

When your back hurts after a long day of standing, simply lying on your side and pulling your knees to your chest will often relieve backache by tilting your pelvis.

Doctors frequently recommend a pelvic-tilting exercise in which you lie flat on your back with your knees bent and both feet flat on the floor so that you can flatten your lower back against the floor with a tail-tucking movement.

Combat the Deterioration of Aging with Good Posture

As you grow older and your intervertebral discs begin to deteriorate, good posture is more important than ever, since over time the pull of gravity can aggravate a tendency to slump. If you have osteoporosis (see Chapter 4), habitual slumping can cause progressive compression of softened vertebrae—until the upper spine collapses into a "dowager's hump."

Young people who are successful in maintaining good posture throughout the early years of life have a much better chance of avoiding the slump of aging. If you still have youth on your side, be sure to take advantage of the opportunity to cultivate habitually good posture that will last a lifetime.

The Special Problems of Sitting

Most of us would rather sit that stand. Yet, if you have a low-back problem, you might be able to stand more comfortably than sit. Scientific studies have shown that there is more pressure on the lower spine when sitting than when standing. When you sit with your lower back unsupported, for example, pressure on the lumbar discs is increased by 40 percent. This means that if you weigh 120 pounds and there is a pressure of 70 pounds on your lower spine when you stand, this pressure is increased to about 100 pounds when you sit in a slumped posture. If you weigh 200 pounds, the pressure on your lumbar discs during unsupported sitting increases to 170 pounds. If you lean forward, the pressure increases even more.

Obviously, if you have a lumbar disc problem, you have to avoid excessive sitting. When you do sit, you should be careful to sit properly.

Solving Driver's Backache

What do you do about backache caused by a bad car seat? Ask Horace T., a traveling salesman who has a chronic disc problem. "My back used to be so painful after a long trip that I could hardly get out of my car," Horace recalled. "When I learned how to support my lower back while sitting, my back trouble practically disappeared."

When Horace sat in his car, he moved his car seat forward enough to enable him to reach the gas and brake pedals while sitting with his knees comfortably bent. (People with sciatica should avoid stretching their legs out in front in order to avoid stretching the sciatic nerve.) Horace also scooted all the way back in his car seat, sat erect, and then placed a paperback book in the small of his back. The erect posture and the support were enough to prevent his lumbar spine from slumping, thus avoiding excessive pressure on his lumbar discs.

If you travel a lot and your back bothers you, try supporting your lower back with a paperback book and see if that helps. If the support feels good, you can pin a hand towel around the book for padding and suspend the wrapped book over the back of your car seat with a couple pieces of string. Hang the book so that it stays at just the right level to support your lumbar curve (the small of your back) when you get into your car.

Selecting the Proper Chair

For prolonged sitting, the type of chair you select can be very important, even when you have good sitting posture.

Whenever possible, it's always best to sit in a firmly padded straight-back chair that has armrests. Sitting with your forearms on an armrest and your upper spine supported in a slightly reclining position will reduce stress on your spine and relieve tension on your muscles, especially if you sit with your lower back supported just enough to maintain your normal lumbar curve.

If you don't have any lower back support when you sit, you should make a conscious effort to sit erect and maintain a slight arch in your lower back. Of course, when you sit erect and unsupported, there is more tension on your muscles. But remember that when your spine slumps, there is pressure on your vertebrae as well as on your discs. If you happen to have spinal arthritis or osteoporosis, pressure on your vertebrae from slumping can irritate arthritic spurs and compress softened vertebrae. Even if you have a strong, healthy back and spine, bad sitting postures can cause backache simply by straining joints and ligaments. So it's important to cultivate good sitting posture as well as good standing posture.

Enhance Good Sitting Posture with Proper Chair Height

Even when your sitting posture is good, the height of your chair should be considered. If your chair is too low, excessive bending of your knees and hips will tend to encourage slumping of your spine. If your chair is too high,

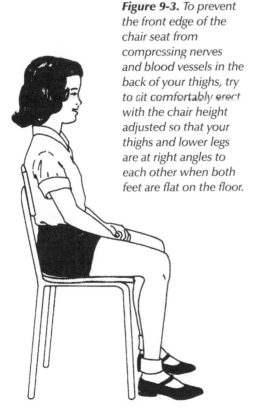

Figure 9-3. To prevent the front edge of the chair seat from compressing nerves and blood vessels in the back of your thighs, try to sit comfortably erect with the chair height adjusted so that your thighs and lower legs are at right angles to each other when both feet are flat on the floor.

so that your feet do not rest freely on the floor, the pressure of the front edge of the chair seat against the back of your thighs will irritate nerves and interfere with blood flow, causing numbness, swelling, and weakness in your feet and ankles. (Prolonged sitting with your legs crossed can cause weakness in one foot by placing pressure against nerves behind the knee.)

When you must sit at a desk or at a workbench for hours at a time, select a chair that allows you to sit comfortably with your knees a little higher than your hips while your feet are flat on the floor. Most office chairs can be adjusted in height to suit your leg length. Some may even have an adjustable back support.

A seat cushion can be used when a chair is too low. When a chair is too high and is not adjustable, it might be necessary to place a platform under your feet. Or, if your chair is made of wood, you may simply saw an inch or two off the chair legs. Do whatever you have to do to keep your spine from slumping and to keep the pressure off the back of your thighs.

If you have back trouble, the most important thing to remember in finding a chair that is suitable for you is to find one that feels *comfortable* to you. Since there are many types of back trouble, the type of chair that feels good to one back patient might not feel good to another. You should, of course, always try to observe the rules of good sitting posture when using a chair of any type.

How to Protect Your Spine with Proper Lifting Techniques

We all know that it's best to squat and keep your spine as vertical as possible when lifting. Simply leaning forward tends to strain the spine by placing leverage on the lower back. When you lean forward and lift a weight, the leverage and the strain are greatly increased. Bending forward 20 degrees and picking up a 44-pound weight, for example, more than *doubles* the pressure on your lower back and spinal discs. The strain is even greater if you attempt to lift a weight while sitting. Twisting while leaning forward and lifting (while standing or sitting) will further increase the risk of injury.

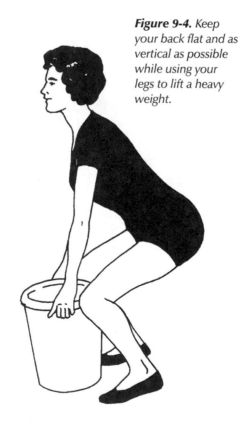

Figure 9-4. Keep your back flat and as vertical as possible while using your legs to lift a heavy weight.

Obviously, if you want to protect your spine from strain, you should cultivate the habit of lifting properly. And all lifting should be done from a *standing* position. To do this, you'll have to keep your spine as vertical as you can and then squat down so that you can lift close to your body. This will enable you to lift with your legs rather than with your back.

Whenever possible, start your lifting about two feet off the floor so that you don't have to bend over so far. Always hold heavy objects close to your body when you carry them. If necessary, wear an apron to prevent soiling of your clothing.

Keep Your Legs Strong!

In order to lift properly, *your leg muscles must be strong enough to permit you to do a full squat.* It will be necessary, therefore, to do squatting exercises regularly to keep your legs strong. If you have weak legs, you'll be forced to bend over to lift a weight from the floor, thus endangering your spine.

If you cannot do several unassisted squats, you should begin doing squatting exercises today!

Don't Reach Out and Lift

Even if your legs are strong, you could easily strain your back by leaning forward and extending your arms out in front to lift something. Leaning over a table to raise a window, for example, or reaching into the trunk of your car to remove a spare tire may place so much leverage on your lower back that you could suffer a severe strain. You may be especially vulnerable to strain if your back muscles are weak or if your spine is unstable because of a mechanical abnormality.

Keeping your back muscles strong will help protect against strain, but strong muscles will not protect unstable joints and ligaments from strain during awkward movements or unbalanced exertion. So while it's important to keep your muscles strong, it's equally important to use your arms, back, and legs in the most mechanically efficient way possible. All it takes is a little common sense to avoid placing excessive leverage on your arms and your back.

Push Instead of Pull

Just as lifting an object out in front with your arms or while bending over can strain your back with excessive leverage, *pulling* on an object might also strain your back with improper leverage.

When you are moving heavy furniture or some other bulky object, it's usually better to *push* rather than pull. In order to push correctly, you should straighten your spine and lean toward the object so that you can push with your legs. This way, as in proper lifting, your legs instead of your back will bear most of the load.

Try to *push in line with your spine* as much as possible.

When you are forced to pull on an object, lean backward so that you can push with your legs (in line with your spine), thus avoiding the leverage that would be placed on your spine by pulling with your arms.

How Parnell C. Relieved His Back Pain by Using Proper Lifting Techniques

Parnell C. was a busy plumber with a long history of recurring back pain. When he was referred to my office for treatment of an on-the-job injury, I found that he had a spinal structural abnormality, predisposing him to back strain. Injury usually occurred only when he lifted in positions that placed him at a mechanical disadvantage—when he was under a house or while installing a tub, for example.

I told Parnell how to brace his elbows on his knees when he was lifting an object while kneeling and how to brace with one arm in order to lift or pull with the opposite arm. When he learned how to avoid placing leverage on his spine during exertion, he got along fine.

"I just did not realize how important it is to protect my spine from leverage when using my arms," Parnell confessed. "I haven't had any more back trouble since you told me how to lift properly."

If you have structural instability in your lower spine because of a mechanical abnormality, as Parnell did, you'll have to make a special effort to protect your spine from excessive leverage. None of us can always avoid awkward positions that might cause slipping of the lower lumbar vertebrae. But if you cultivate the habit of lifting properly and try to avoid mechanically inefficient exertion, your chances of suffering a low-back strain will be greatly reduced, even if you have an unstable spine.

Once you understand how to use your arms, legs, and back properly, you'll be able to perform more work as well as protect your back from strain.

How to Protect Your Back with Proper Sleeping Postures

Most of us spend more than one-third of our life in bed. And we do so gladly. When we finish a long, hard day at work or at play, flopping into bed is pure luxury. A good night's sleep restores our reserves for another day—provided, of course, that we sleep well without interruption.

Unfortunately, a bad sleeping posture, like a bad sitting or standing posture, can have an adverse effect on your spine. The result may be a chronic back problem that interferes with sleep at night and then nags you during the day. So it's just as important to pay as much attention to your sleeping posture as to your sitting posture.

Begin with a Good Mattress

As you learned in Chapter 4, a good, firm mattress is absolutely essential for bed rest without backache. A mattress that sags places a strain on joints, ligaments, and muscles. A bed that's too hard might cause backache by failing to conform to the natural curves of the body. Obviously, before you can do much about improving your sleeping posture, you'll have to make sure that you have a good mattress.

If you think your mattress might be too soft but you're not sure, try placing your mattress on the floor for one night to see if you rest better. If the extra firmness seems to help, you should buy a new mattress set—or you may place a half-inch-thick sheet of plywood between your mattress and your springs.

Sleeping on Your Back Is Usually Best

Generally, the best way to sleep is to lie flat on your back. And it's usually best to use a thin pillow. But if you have a hump in your back, you may have to use a thicker pillow to keep your head from tilting too far back. If you have low-back trouble, sciatica, or short hip flexors, you may also have to place a pillow under your knees so that you can rest with your knees and your hips slightly bent. This will relieve a pull on your hamstrings and sciatic nerve and allow your pelvis to tilt back a little so that your lumbar spine will rest flat on the mattress.

Don't use foam rubber pillows. Such pillows are too springy to provide solid support for your head and neck. Whenever possible, choose a good feather or down pillow.

Side Posture Sleeping Is Okay

Many people find that sleeping on their side is the most comfortable position of all, since this position allows a greater amount of pelvic tilting with bent knees. The position that is most comfortable for you—on your back or on your side—will depend upon what kind of back trouble you have, your body size, the condition of your muscles, and other factors. If you have a hip problem, it might be necessary to place a pillow between your knees when you sleep on your side. People with shoulder arthritis might find it impossible to lie on one side. When a mattress is very hard, sleeping on one side might interfere with the circulation of blood in the arm being compressed, causing the arm to "go to sleep."

Obviously, there is no single sleeping posture that everyone can use. You may have to experiment in order to find a sleeping posture that suits you best. Try to avoid sleeping face down.

No matter what sleeping posture you assume, you'll change positions several times during the night, even when sleeping soundly. Chances are you'll roll over on your side occasionally, thus relieving tension on muscles and joints and aiding circulation. It's better to move around in bed than to stay in one position. (Clogging of arteries occurs most often during bed rest at night when circulation slows from inactivity and blood fat is high from an evening meal. So it's okay to roll around in bed when you sleep.)

Try to Break the Habit of Sleeping Face Down

I often hear patients say that the only way they can sleep is in a facedown position, that is, on their abdomen. Many of these people do sleep well facedown—until they begin to have back or neck trouble caused by injury or aging. Once arthritis begins to develop in your spine, for example, sleeping facedown tends to jam sensitive joints together. Turning your head to one side may irritate arthritic joints in your neck. Damaging pressure might also be placed on your temporomandibular (TMJ) joints, especially after you lose some of your teeth and your bite changes due to malocclusion.

Even if you presently sleep well lying facedown, you should begin making an effort to break the habit so that you can sleep on your back or on your side. With time and aging, there may come a day when arthritic changes in your back, neck, and shoulders will make it difficult or impossible to sleep facedown without interruption by pain. If such a bad sleeping posture is a deeply ingrained habit, it might take months of fitful sleep to break the habit. This can be a real problem if you suddenly develop back trouble. So it might be a good idea to begin now to cultivate the habit of sleeping on your back or on your side—before a facedown position begins to become uncomfortable.

Special Advice for Stomach Sleepers

When you do sleep on your abdomen, you probably should not use a pillow, since this might force excessive extension or arching of your spine.

Simply lying facedown on a soft, saggy mattress will extend your spine too much. Using a pillow in such a position may be the straw that breaks the camel's back. If you do use a pillow, it should be thin.

If you must lie on your abdomen, you should at least make sure that you have a good, firm mattress that does not sag. Even then, it might be a good idea to turn onto your side enough to permit you to bend one leg, thus tilting your pelvis a little. You may then use a thin pillow without arching your spine.

As in sitting postures, there is no one sleeping posture that suits everyone. If you have arthritis in your spinal joints, a bulging disc, or a spinal deformity, sleeping facedown or on one side might be so uncomfortable or painful that you won't be able to maintain such a position for very long.

As a general rule, painful sleeping postures should always be avoided. In certain types of back injuries, however, as in spinal fractures, your doctor might recommend that you lie on your abdomen or that you assume some other normally uncomfortable sleeping posture.

Persons with ankylosing spondylitis (see Chapter 8), a disease in which the affected spinal joints fuse together, may not always be allowed to assume the most comfortable sleeping posture. It might be necessary to sleep flat on your back (without a pillow under the knees) or even on your abdomen, to keep your spine as straight as possible while fusion of your vertebrae is taking place. You might not even be allowed to use a pillow under your head or to turn your head to one side when you sleep on your back. Your doctor might prescribe special medication so that you can endure the discomfort of sleeping with your spine straight, lest you gradually change your sleeping posture to a more comfortable (but more harmful) position as fusion and deformity progresses. You should, of course, be under the care of a rheumatologist who can help you avoid the flexion (forward bending) deformity of ankylosing spondylitis.

Relieve Back Pain with Bed Breaks

It's always a good idea to lie down occasionally to relieve the pressures on your spine, especially when you have a backache. You don't have to sleep to benefit from bed rest. When your back is fatigued and aching, simply lying down will allow compressed discs to expand, pushing the vertebrae apart enough to relieve jamming and overriding of joint surfaces. Otherwise, a buildup of pain may trigger muscle spasm, which can lock you into a painful posture.

At the end of a long day on your feet, you may be as much as three-quarters of an inch shorter in height as a result of the intervertebral discs being squeezed by the pull of gravity and the weight of your body. This can result in bulging of weak discs as well as irritation of spinal joints. Much of this can be relieved simply by lying down two or three times a day whenever possible.

Lying on a slant board with your feet anchored at the high end of the board will further relieve pressure and expand joints by providing a little stretch on your spine. One business executive I know keeps a slant board in his office for daily use. "Lying upside down on my slant board for a few minutes a day not only relieves my backache but also refreshes my mind," he maintains.

One thing is certain: It's difficult to think clearly when you have a backache. It may be safe to say, therefore, that if you have backaches, you might be able to improve your mind by improving your posture!

Postural Hypotension

Postural hypotension—or feeling dizzy when you stand abruptly from a sitting or reclining position—really has nothing to do with bad posture. If you experience this symptom, however, you should see your doctor. Failure of your vascular system to maintain blood pressure after sudden changes in posture might indicate low blood pressure, loss of body fluid, overmedication for high blood pressure, or some other problem that might need attention. Most of the time, however, postural hypotension is not a serious problem. Just make sure that you don't jump out of bed or get out of a chair too quickly and risk falling because of sudden dizziness.

Ergonomics: Posture Problems at Work

With seventy-five million Americans using computers at work and at home, computer-related neck pain, headache, upper back myofascitis, carpal tunnel syndrome, and other work-related ailments are increasing in direct proportion to changing work stress. Ergonomics, the study of conditions in the work place, is fast developing into a field specializing in the prevention of injuries caused by repetitive trauma and bad postures.

With the advent of computers and electronic office machines, prolonged sitting while watching a screen and operating a keyboard has resulted in an increase in back pain and other joint problems that are not typical of the usual postural strains. Carpal tunnel syndrome, for example, an irritation of the median nerve in the wrist, causing numbness and weakness in the hand, has become common as a result of repetitive and prolonged hand and wrist action over a keyboard.

Sitting hour after hour watching a computer screen while entering data electronically has resulted in a variety of aches and pains involving the neck, shoulders, low back, hips, and thighs. In order to reduce strain and repetitive trauma, it is essential to make sure that your sitting posture is good. The correct chair height will allow you to sit erect with both feet flat and your thighs parallel to the floor, without excessive pressure on the back of your thighs. Your keyboard should be at a level that will permit you to work with your forearms parallel to the floor. And to avoid sitting with your head

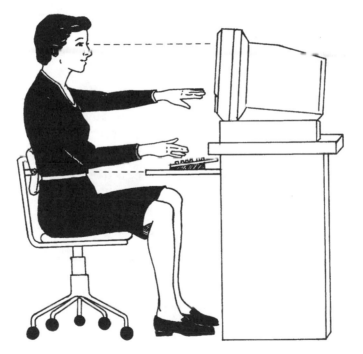

Figure 9-5. The increasing use of computers at home and on the job requires special attention to sitting postures in order to avoid repetitive trauma aches and pains.

turned and your spine tilted, screens should be placed so that you can look straight ahead as much as possible.

When your job forces you to sit or stand in one position for a long time, you should take frequent breaks and move around to relieve strain and to stimulate blood flow.

Many large offices and industries try to design the workplace so that employees can work efficiently and with as little strain as possible. Some job stresses are unavoidable, however. Static postures and repetitive movements must be countered with frequent exercise or rest breaks, and you should make a special effort to make sure that your work postures are comfortable. If you sit, for example, find a chair that's best for you. Make sure that you are able to sit in an upright posture with your arms at a comfortable level and your work directly in front of you. If you work at a bench, find one that's waist high. During prolonged standing, placing one foot up on a stool might relieve back strain. Don't ever work in postures that require you to lean or hold your arms up high. Use common sense. Practicing good ergonomics includes using correct lifting postures, avoiding fatigue, and many of the self-help measures discussed in this book. With good working postures, you'll feel better, be more productive, and be injured less frequently—and you'll also be more valued as an employee.

SUMMARY

1. The delicately balanced spinal curves that allow upright posture and the use of your hands must be protected by proper posture while standing, sitting, and lying down.

2. Bad posture can cause backache and other symptoms by placing a strain on muscles, joints, ligaments, and discs, resulting in arthritis, disc degeneration, nerve root irritation, and other problems.

3. Good standing posture is best maintained simply by developing the habit of standing tall.

4. Backache caused by standing at work can often be relieved by placing one foot up on a low box to produce a slight pelvic tilt.

5. Excessive pressure on the lumbar discs when sitting can be relieved by sitting erect or by supporting the lower back enough to maintain the normal lumbar curve.

6. When you lift an object, always squat down and keep your spine as vertical as possible so that you lift with your legs and not with your back.

7. Don't ever lean forward and lift with your arms out in front!

8. It's always better to push than to pull, and you should lean toward the object you're pushing so that you can push in line with your spine.

9. Sleeping on your back or on your side places less strain on your spine than sleeping on your abdomen.

10. The most comfortable sitting, standing, or sleeping posture is generally best for persons who have a specific back or neck problem—except in the case of persons suffering from a spinal fracture or ankylosing spondylitis.

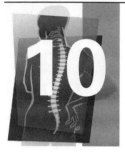

Preventing and Easing Back Pain During Pregnancy

You learned in Chapter 4 that 10 pounds of potbelly centered 10 inches out in front of the spine requires a 50-pound pull in lower back muscles to maintain an erect posture. This places an extra 50 pounds of pressure on the lower spine. And when body weight increases, pressure on the lumbar discs increases greatly.

Weight gain as a result of obesity usually takes place over a period of years, allowing the body to compensate somewhat for gradual and uneven accumulation of weight. When a woman becomes pregnant, however, weight gain is rapid, averaging about 19 pounds in nine months. After several months, there may be 10 or 12 pounds of out-front weight that places an unaccustomed load on low-back muscles. This increase in abdominal weight shifts the center of gravity forward, forcing the individual to lean backward in order to balance body weight. Such overloading of lumbar (spina erecta) muscles results in an inflamed and aching back after periods of standing or exertion.

As pregnancy progresses, the body produces a hormone called "relaxin," which relaxes sacroiliac and pubic ligaments so that the pelvis can expand as needed for delivery of the baby. The abdominal muscles also relax and stretch as the abdomen enlarges.

As a result of all these unaccustomed changes in body weight, muscles, joints, and ligaments, back trouble is almost inevitable. In addition to fatigue and aching in muscles that support the spine, spinal joints may be jammed and irritated. Compression on weak lumbar discs may cause some of them to bulge. Sacroiliac strain may occur when sudden or prolonged torsion is placed on relaxed and vulnerable ligaments. There is much that you can do to prevent or minimize back pain associated with pregnancy, however. This chapter offers a program that can be followed before, during, and after pregnancy.

Prenatal Prevention Measures

Everything you have learned in other chapters of this book—about posture, lifting techniques, home treatment for muscle and joint pain, and so on—will help in easing the back pain associated with pregnancy. It may be more important, however, to make an effort to *prevent* back pain by taking meas-

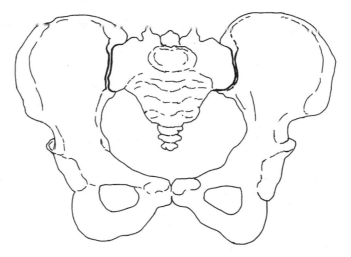

Figure 10-1. The basin of a female pelvis is wider than that of a male pelvis. The sacroiliac joints, which join the ilia on each side, relax during birth to allow further expansion of the pelvis.

ures beforehand. Once weak back muscles have been overloaded by the off-centered weight of pregnancy and the sacroiliac ligaments have been strained by improper lifting and sitting postures, the resulting muscle, joint, and ligament pain can be chronic and debilitating. The exercises described in other chapters of this book would be helpful in preparing for pregnancy and during early pregnancy when there is no back pain. The simple, basic exercises described in this chapter, however, would be adequate and may be done throughout pregnancy if they do not cause pain.

If you are planning or expecting a pregnancy, what you learn in this chapter can make the difference between going about business as usual or hobbling around in fear of pain.

Preparing for Pregnancy with Exercise

This simple exercise program should begin before you become pregnant. You may continue doing the exercises during and after pregnancy. Remember that the better shape you're in when you give birth, the easier the delivery will be and the faster you'll recover. Begin these exercises with light and comfortable movements. Gradually, increase the amount of exercise you do over a period of several weeks. Go by the way you feel. Don't do any exercise that is painful or uncomfortable.

For the Abdominal Muscles

The pelvic tilt: Lie on your back with your knees bent and both feet flat on the floor. Contract your abdominal muscles so that your lower back is flattened against the floor and your pelvis is tilted upward, as in pelvic thrusting. Do this ten times or more every day.

Leg raising: Lie on your back with one leg bent (foot on the floor) and the other leg straight out and flat on the floor. Raise the straight leg to about 45 degrees several times. Repeat this movement with each leg five or six times.

For the Low-Back Muscles

Leg pointing exercise: Begin on your hands and knees. Straighten one leg and lift it to 90 degrees (parallel to the floor) several times, as if pointing at the wall with your foot. Exercise both legs equally. As pregnancy progresses, this exercise can be done without any uncomfortable strain on the abdomen, and it tends to place a corrective rotation on the sacroiliac joint.

Half squat: Hold on to a bed post and squat halfway down several times, keeping both feet flat on the floor in order to activate buttock and low-back muscles. You can use the bedpost for assistance in keeping your balance and to assist your thigh muscles until your legs become strong enough to squat unassisted. Flat-footed squats strengthen and shape buttock muscles as well as thigh muscles.

Walk regularly: Simple walking, indoors or outside, will condition your cardiovascular and respiratory systems as well as tone the body's major muscle groups.

Relieving Back Pain During Pregnancy

Not every woman has back pain during pregnancy, but enough do to warrant a special effort to begin exercising several months before pregnancy begins. When back pain does occur, it usually begins after the first trimester (after the first three months). Pain may be worse in the final few months when the abdomen is larger and there is more arching in the lower spine. Use of high-heeled shoes during this time will increase arching of the lower back, further increasing the load on lumbar muscles and jamming joints on the back of the spine. Make sure that you have a good pair of low-heeled walking shoes that are cushioned and properly fitted.

As the months pass and the abdomen enlarges, it may be necessary to lie on one side while resting, sleeping, or making love. You don't have to give up the pleasures of sex just because you are pregnant. You'll learn in Chapter 13 about sexual postures that will protect your back while adding variety and pleasure to lovemaking. If you have a history of miscarriage, your doctor might advise against the penetration of sexual intercourse during the first three months of pregnancy. Masturbation and other techniques can be used to relieve sexual tension.

Simple moist heat and massage (Chapter 4) applied over back muscles can provide welcome relief for a tired and aching back. Lying on one side and pulling the knees up a little to round out the lower back will often relieve backache that occurs after prolonged standing. If you have pain across your lower back, with symptoms indicating a lumbar or lumbosacral strain, you can be fitted with a special corset designed to support your back as well as lift your abdomen. Such corsets shift the center of gravity backward a little to relieve strain on back muscles. You should not take any kind of pain medication without your doctor's permission.

Stretch the Spine a Little

Because of the increased load that pregnancy places on the spinal discs in the lower back, it might be a good idea to stretch the spine a little each day. Simply lying down will help reduce pressure on the intervertebral discs. But when there is painful bulging of a bad lumbar disc, traction or stretching will sometimes bring relief by allowing gravity to decompress the disc enough to retract the bulge.

Hanging from a tree limb or a chinning bar might be helpful if it can be done while both feet remain on the ground. Probably the best gravity-

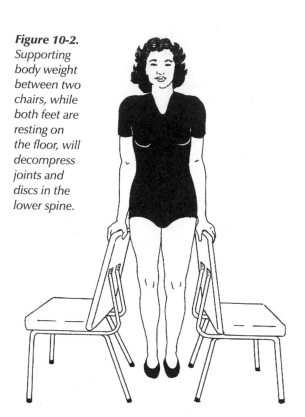

Figure 10-2. Supporting body weight between two chairs, while both feet are resting on the floor, will decompress joints and discs in the lower spine.

assisted traction to use during pregnancy is to support your weight between two chairs turned back to back. Be sure to keep both feet on the floor so that the weight on your arms and the stretch on your back can be controlled by support from your feet.

For simple loosening of your vertebrae, try doing the camel-horse exercise shown in Chapter 5. Begin on your hands and knees and simply arch your back up and down several times.

Postpartum Problems

In many cases, back pain begins *after* the baby has been delivered—in the postpartum period. All the bending, lifting, bathing, changing and washing diapers, and so on, repeated many times day and night, is a job for a well-conditioned athlete. An unprepared and physically unfit first-time mother with a newborn baby can hardly endure such a load. Overwork, along with poor sitting and standing postures and improper lifting techniques, tends to strain weakened sacroiliac ligaments as well as back muscles, causing acute debilitating back pain.

Make sure that you have a special table for bathing and dressing your baby—a table high enough to allow you to work without bending over. Always lift and hold your baby close to your body in order to reduce leverage on your lower back and sacroiliac joints. Never reach out and lift your baby with your arms extended; a sudden shoulder or back pain may cause you to drop the baby. If you have shoulder tendonitis (see Chapter 3) or a lower back problem, lifting a baby out of a deep crib can be a real problem.

In the case of tendonitis, it might be helpful to brace your elbows against the inside of the crib so that you can lift your baby by bending your elbows, thus reducing leverage on your shoulders. If you have back pain, don't lean forward while holding a baby. Keep the baby close to you and squat with your spine as upright as possible when placing the baby on a low surface.

Always carry your baby close to your body. If necessary, wear an apron so that you don't have to worry about being soiled by wet or dirty diapers.

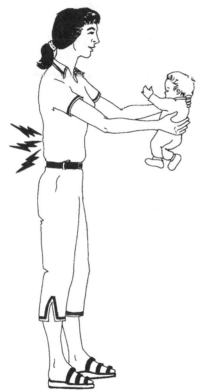

Figure 10-3. Never hold a baby or any weight with the arms extended in front. Doing so places damaging leverage on the lower back.

Remember to sit and stand erect so that your weight is centered over your pelvis. Sitting in a slumped posture tends to shift weight to the back of your pelvis, placing a rotating strain on weak sacroiliac ligaments.

A "baby carrier" designed to carry a baby in front or in back, worn much like a backpack, can be purchased through any major department store. Generally, there is less strain placed on the spine if you carry the baby in back. You can experiment with such a carrier to determine what is most comfortable for you—or you may simply use a baby carriage if that works best.

When Sacroiliac Strain Occurs

A sacroiliac strain is characterized by pain on one side of the buttock area, with increased pain when you bear weight on that side, causing a noticeable limp. Your doctor might test for sacroiliac strain by raising one leg straight up until pain is caused by forced rotation in the sensitive joint. You can find the sacroiliac joints by locating the dimples on the back of your pelvis. Pain resulting from thumb pressure applied over one of these dimples may be an indication of a sacroiliac problem.

It's important to avoid postural strains that place leverage on the sacroiliac joints, especially when one of the joints has been strained. Always sit erect so that you have a little arch in your lower back. A paperback book or a folded hand towel placed in the small of your lower back will reduce rotation in the sacroiliac joints, whether you're sitting at home or in a car.

Everyone, especially a new mother, should avoid reaching out to lift something. Lifting a bag of groceries out of the trunk of a car or leaning over to raise a window, for example, places so much leverage on the lower back that it would be quite easy to strain the postpartum sacroiliac joints.

Sacroiliac Support

When a sacroiliac strain is bad enough to affect movement, a sacroiliac belt might help. This is a strap that encircles the pelvis to clamp down and tighten the sacroiliac joints. There may be a pad on the back of the strap for placement over the sacrum. This pad can be removed if it causes discomfort. If you remember what you learned in Chapter 4, you know that a sacroiliac belt is different from a lumbar or lumbosacral support. So be sure to ask for a sacroiliac belt.

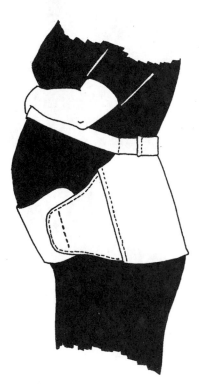

Figure 10-4. When there is low-back pain during pregnancy, a doctor might prescribe a special maternity corset that supports the abdomen as well as the lower back.

In rare cases, a sacroiliac joint might bind or lock, causing acute pain during certain movements. A single manipulation by a chiropractor, osteopath, orthopedist, physiatrist, or physical therapist will sometimes unlock the joint and restore mobility. If a sacroiliac strain is bad enough to warrant wearing a sacroiliac belt, check with an orthopedist to first determine if you have a locked joint, or, as the doctor would say, "loss of congruity in the joint."

Backache Relief with Moist Heat and Massage

No matter what you might do to prepare for pregnancy and prevent back pain, it is almost inevitable that you will experience a backache at some point during a pregnancy. The camel-horse exercise described in Chapter 5, in which you arch your back up and down several times while you are on your hands and knees, is a good way to warm up your muscles and loosen your spine. Several minutes of moist heat applied over your back, followed by a few minutes of kneading or stroking of the muscles on each side of your spine, will also do wonders in relieving backache. Such treatment will be more effective and much safer than most physical therapy modalities (a physical therapist might decline using ultrasound, diathermy, or electrical stimulation over the back of a pregnant woman).

As your pregnancy progresses, it may be difficult to lie facedown for a back massage. Try lying over pillows or cushions so as to create a space for your abdomen. Have someone place a moist-heat heating pad over the aching portion of your back. You can purchase a special insulated heating pad with a cloth cover that can be moistened under a faucet. After the heating pad is removed, have someone knead or stroke your back muscles from bottom to top. Any kind of oil or skin cream can be used as a lubricant.

If your abdomen is too large for you to be able to lie facedown, you can lie on your side and strap the heating pad to your back. Following an application of heat, while you are still lying on your side, your mate can massage your back muscles. This simple procedure will be more effective than a visit to a spa, and it can be used as often as needed.

Keep in Touch with Your Doctor

Backache that is persistent or accompanied by fever should always be brought to the attention of an obstetrician or a family physician. Kidney problems, infection, disc herniation, and other problems must be ruled out before depending solely upon home remedies. Remember, however, that spinal X rays should not be made during the first three or four months of pregnancy. An X-ray exam is sometimes done in the final trimester (last three months) of pregnancy if a contracted pelvis (small pelvic outlet) is suspected. Otherwise, X-ray or CAT scan radiation should be avoided if possible.

SUMMARY

1. Preparation for pregnancy should begin with an exercise program that starts several months before pregnancy begins.

2. Without strong back muscles, back pain is more likely to occur when the center of gravity moves forward as pregnancy progresses.

3. Wearing high-heeled shoes increases arching of the lumbar spine, adding to back pain by jamming spinal joints.

4. In the final trimester of pregnancy and in the postpartum period, relaxed sacroiliac ligaments are easily strained by bad posture and improper lifting technique.

5. During pregnancy, low-back pain can often be relieved by wearing a special corset that lifts the abdomen while it supports the lower back.

6. You should have a special table for bathing and clothing your baby so that you won't have to work in a bent-over position.

7. Try not to lean over and reach out with your arms to lift your baby or any other object; you could strain a weak sacroiliac joint.

8. A sacroiliac strain can sometimes be helped by wearing a sacroiliac belt.

9. In the later months of pregnancy, it might be necessary to lie on one side while resting, sleeping, or making love.

10. Moist heat, massage, and gravity-assisted traction might be helpful in relieving back pain caused by inflamed muscles or a bulging disc.

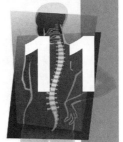

How to Protect a Painful Back During Sex and while Pregnant

One evening around 8:00 P.M. I received a telephone call from **John D.**, a middle-aged patient who had chronic back pain. "I'm in trouble, Doc," he began. "I was having sex and my back locked up. I can't move, and one of my legs is hanging off the bed."

I was familiar with John's history, and I knew that overexertion in a bad posture had wrenched a diseased joint and triggered a locking muscle spasm. I advised John to call an ambulance and go to the emergency room for medication if he wanted pain relief that would allow him to move about. He could then have his wife drive him home. "I can't do that," John explained. "I'm with a girlfriend, and my wife thinks I'm out of town on business."

Obviously, John was in a tough spot. I told him to take a couple of aspirin and put a cold pack over the painful area of his back. He could then either lie on his side with a pillow between his knees or on his back with a pillow under his knees. I explained that by morning, when the acute pain has subsided, he should be able to get up and move around. He called my office the next morning and jubilantly reported that he was much better and planned to spend a few more days with his girlfriend.

John never learns. He had a chronic back problem that could hardly withstand the unaccustomed exertion and the unfamiliar postures of an illicit love affair with a young woman. There was, however, much that he could do to protect his back and prevent back pain during sex, primarily involving moderation and sexual postures.

Much of what I told John about how to relieve his pain has been discussed in other chapters of this book (see Chapter 4). In this chapter, I'll explain how sexual postures affect your back, how to prevent back pain during sex, and how to have sex while back pain is present. I gave John a few tips on how he could have sex without irritating or overloading an unstable spinal joint. The advice was apparently helpful, because he reported a few days later that he had had "a successful rendezvous."

The Benefits of a Healthy Sex Life

Sex is a driving life force we all happily contend with. It is one of life's free and healthful pleasures. Because nature has instilled this need to assure perpetuation of the species, expression and performance of sex has beneficial physiological effects. Regular sex fulfills a need and an evolutionary purpose that fits in with nature's design for the cycle of life. The nervous explosion of an orgasm triggers release of hormones that provide temporary relief from mental and physical pain. As long as there is sexual activity, hormonal influences tend to keep the organism young so that life will be prolonged for continued reproduction. When sexual activity is discontinued, nature may interpret this as a signal that there is no longer a reason for survival of the individual. Health and vitality may then begin to decline. What it all comes down to is that we need regular sex to keep hormones flowing for a longer, happier, and healthier life.

Stress-Free Sex Combats Aging, Prolongs Life, and Eases Back Pain

A 1999 survey reported that the average American has sex 132 times a year. The worldwide average was 96 times a year. Don't put yourself or your partner into the stressful position of trying to have sex a certain number of times, however. Just try to have sex as often as possible when it is consenting and pleasurable.

According to a January 2001 online HealthScout report, there is evidence to indicate that good, regular sex can make you look younger. A Scottish researcher, for example, who interviewed 3,500 European and American men and women, concluded that making love three times a week can make you look ten years younger! But the sex should be with a regular, compatible partner. The stress and worry of casual sex or marital infidelity might actually *cause* premature aging.

Regular sex, like regular exercise, can help reduce body weight by burning fat. It can also help relieve back pain by stimulating the brain's production of pain-relieving endorphins. Release of testosterone and growth hormones during an orgasm strengthens bones and muscles and boosts the immune system. So be sure to include regular, stress-free sex in your exercise and treatment programs.

Age Is No Excuse for Celibacy

The literature suggests that the more often you have sex, the more likely you will continue to enjoy sex at an advanced age. Age-related infirmities and body aches and pains often require adjustments in methods of having sex. But there is every reason to believe that sex should be enjoyed by anyone who is able to have sex, no matter what the age of the person.

When I visit nursing homes, my heart goes out to the elderly residents who still have sexual desires but are suddenly placed in an environment with no privacy and no opportunity to engage in sex with a partner. I recall the heartbreaking scene of a disabled couple, both in wheelchairs, who spent hours holding hands while parked in a secluded but public corner of a nursing home recreation room with no place to go to consummate their love.

The point is, it is necessary as well as healthful to have sex as long as desire and ability are present. No matter how old you are or what kind of disability you might have, you should have sex as often as you want it. Unrelieved sexual tension is unhealthy as well as disconcerting.

Unlike exercise and eating, it is not possible to get too much sex—unless, like John, you overload a bad back. When a sexual urge is satisfied, the desire for sex simply disappears for a while.

Satisfying a frequent sexual urge has no harmful effects and will, in fact, provide beneficial hormonal and cardiovascular effects that improve health and prolong life.

The Special Problems of Pregnancy and Menopause

If you are pregnant or a victim of back pain, you can adjust your sexual postures or techniques to continue with an enjoyable sex life. You owe it to yourself, your partner, and your health. When sexual intercourse is not possible for some reason or a partner is not available, there is absolutely nothing wrong with solo masturbation, which some prefer to call "self relief." Orgasm resulting from any form of sexual activity can be beneficial.

In most cases, it is safe to have sexual intercourse throughout your pregnancy. If you have a history of miscarriage, your doctor might advise you to refrain from penetration during the first three months. But if there is no pain, bleeding, leakage of amniotic fluid, or signs of premature labor, penetration can take place as long as it is desired. Remember that the baby is well protected in a womb filled with amniotic fluid and will not normally be affected by the penetration of sexual intercourse. You can also select a sexual posture, such as rear entry, that will reduce depth of penetration. Always talk with your doctor when you feel there is a problem.

Although many women may experience a decrease in sexual desire during the early and latter months of pregnancy, there may be an increase in sexual desire during the second three months (second trimester). Hormonal changes and an increase in blood flow engorge the clitoris and labia with blood, generating signs of sexual excitement, which can and should be relieved in any manner you choose.

Women around the age of menopause who are not currently sexually active but who may potentially resume sexual intercourse with a male friend or a new husband should occasionally include some form of vaginal penetration in their masturbation techniques. Gynecologists have observed that menopausal women who have not had vaginal penetration for many years often have problems resuming sexual intercourse. Lack of stimulation provided by vaginal penetration may lead to thin vaginal walls that are sensitive and easily irritated. This often happens without hormone replacement therapy, but it is much worse without the stimulation of sexual intercourse. As the old adage goes: "Use it or lose it."

The focus of this chapter is to emphasize the importance of sex and to teach back-pain sufferers how to protect their backs while having sex and how to continue having sex during pregnancy. No one should ever say, "Sex is not important, so we'll just forget about it for a while."

Sex with a Bad Back

When back pain occurs, many things happen that may make sexual intercourse difficult. Most commonly, it is the lower back that is at fault.

When there are plans to have sexual intercourse and you have back pain, it might be helpful to take a couple of aspirin and then warm up your lower back beforehand. The camel-horse exercise for relieving back pain that is described in Chapter 5 can also be used to warm up a bad back. You might also want to try lying on your back with your knees bent and doing a pelvic-tilt exercise by contracting your abdominal muscles while lifting your buttocks up from the floor.

Studies have shown that women with low-back pain have more discomfort during sexual intercourse than men do. The most comfortable position was supine (lying on the back) and the most uncomfortable position was prone (lying facedown).

Suggestion No. 1: Any kind of leverage placed on the spine uses the sacral base at the bottom of the spine as a fulcrum. When you lean away from vertical, especially in a forward direction, the amount of leverage exerted on the bottom of the spine is often enough to wrench or pull an unstable or sensitive joint, triggering muscle spasm and buckling the knees. For this reason, you should avoid postures that require you to lean forward while making love.

Suggestion No. 2: An injured spinal joint is often sensitive and unstable. Repeated pelvic thrusting may cause cumulative irritation that may result in pain and spasm later. Try to avoid a lengthy session of sexual intercourse. A little inventive foreplay will reduce the amount of time required to reach a climax, and the injured partner can be careful to keep their body fairly still.

Suggestion No. 3: A bulging or herniated disc will sometimes protrude far enough to impinge upon a spinal nerve, causing leg pain or muscle spasm that pulls the body to one side or the other. Placing increased weight on a bad disc can cause an increase in leg pain or muscle spasm. You should avoid sexual postures in which you must lift or support the weight of your partner.

Suggestion No. 4: Whether a low-back pain is the result of a joint problem or a bulging disc, any activity that requires lifting the thighs up in front will contract the psoas muscles that attach between the femur (thigh bone) and the lumbar vertebrae. This pull on the psoas muscles also pulls on the lower spine. When back pain is acute, any effort to lift up the legs may trigger a protective spasm in back muscles. (Remember John, whose back "locked" while one leg was hanging off the bed?)

Don't lose your head in the throes of sexual ecstasy and attempt to lift your legs or use your legs for leverage in order to get the most out of a sexual encounter—you could end up like John.

Sexual Postures Anyone Can Use

When you have back pain, you should observe all the suggestions above. Don't continue with any kind of movement or posture if it causes pain or discomfort. Even if you are able to complete the act, you may pay for it later and be out of commission for a while. If one position causes discomfort, try another. As a last resort, you can be passive and let your partner do all the work.

The "Missionary Position"

This inaptly named position may be best for two lovers who want to lie face to face and embrace each other while having sex. The person with the back trouble takes the passive position on the bottom, taking care to bend both

Figure 11-1. A male with back pain can be a passive sexual partner while lying on his back, keeping his knees bent a little to ease tension on the psoas muscles.

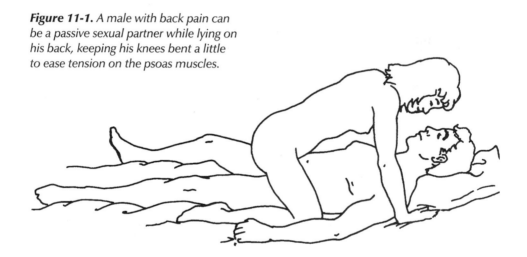

knees a little to relieve pull on the psoas muscles. The person on top may move about in variety of ways, much to the delight of both partners.

The Side Posture Position

A female with back pain or who is pregnant may simply lie on one side with her hips and knees bent (and a pillow between her knees) and allow the male to penetrate her from the back. This position will reduce the depth of penetration, depending upon the degree of pelvic tilt.

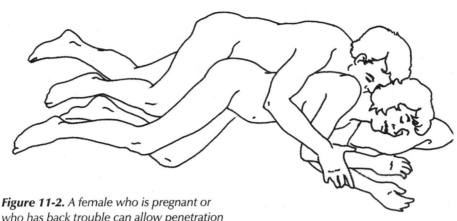

Figure 11-2. A female who is pregnant or who has back trouble can allow penetration from behind in a side posture position.

The "Doggy Position"

This position, in which the female is on her hands and knees while the male penetrates her from behind, can be comfortable for a female who is pregnant or who has back pain. With her weight supported on her hands and knees, her spine is suspended weight-free and there is no pressure on her abdomen. Bent knees and hips eliminate pull on the psoas muscles and the sciatic nerve.

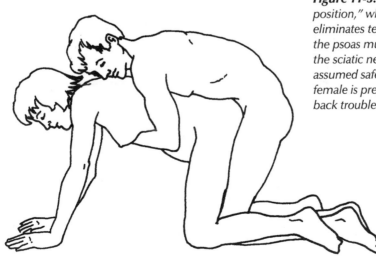

Figure 11-3. The "doggy position," which eliminates tension on the psoas muscles and the sciatic nerve, can be assumed safely when the female is pregnant or has back trouble.

A Supported Pregnancy Position

When a pregnant female wants to lie on her back so that she can see the face of her lover, she can do so in a special supported position. She lies on the edge of her bed with both feet supported by a chair. Her partner, on his

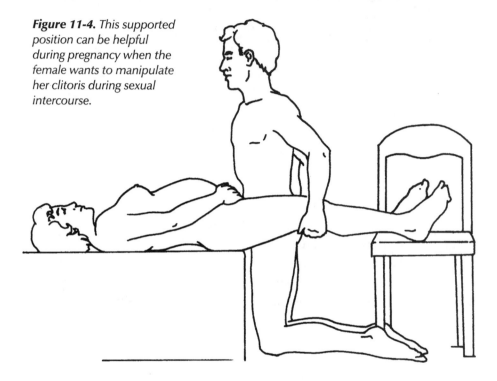

Figure 11-4. This supported position can be helpful during pregnancy when the female wants to manipulate her clitoris during sexual intercourse.

knees between her thighs, lifts her knees a little to reduce tension on her psoas muscles and to prevent arching of her lumbar spine. The female can freely manipulate her clitoris to reach an orgasm during intercourse.

A Bonus in Back-Pain Sex

It is often necessary to proceed cautiously and tenderly with lovemaking when back pain is present. Many couples discover that sex can be more sensual and satisfying when it is done slowly and carefully. And when a special effort is made to help a partner reach an orgasm, whether by mutual masturbation or in sexual intercourse, the satisfaction is greater. Watching a partner enjoy the ecstasy of orgasm is too much to give up, even when you have back pain.

SUMMARY

1. Sexual desire is a natural urge that should be satisfied on a regular basis to assure good health and longevity.

2. When back pain occurs, movements that place leverage on the spine, contract the psoas muscles, or compress the intervertebral discs must be avoided.

3. Generally, the individual who has back pain assumes a passive role while the partner "does all the work."

4. To prevent aggravation of back pain, postures that require leaning over, lifting the legs, or supporting weight should be avoided.

5. Keeping the knees bent and the hip flexed while lying on your back during sex will prevent painful arching of the lumbar spine caused by contraction of the psoas muscles.

6. Don't persist in use of a painful sexual posture; it could be followed by acute pain and muscle spasm.

7. If there is a history of miscarriage, sexual intercourse might be prohibited for the first three months of pregnancy.

8. Special postures can be used to allow sexual intercourse throughout pregnancy, especially a side-posture position that reduces the depth of penetration.

9. Back pain or pregnancy provides an opportunity for a couple to experiment with a variety of methods of making love.

10. Remember the old adage—Use it or lose it. Any approach that will achieve an orgasm that can be shared by a couple is worth the effort.

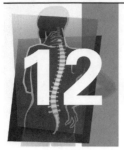

Evaluating Back and Leg Pain after Middle Age

They say that life after retirement is the beginning of the "golden years." This is true for most of us when we are relieved of the stress and responsibility associated with mundane employment and unworthy bosses. What a relief it is to finally walk away from a clock-punching job after spending years counting the days leading to retirement.

Unfortunately, for many of us, the time and hard work that have earned us retirement have also taken a toll on us physically. The cumulative effects of job wear and tear begin to become evident in the years to follow. Our joints begin to stiffen, eyesight dims, and hearing diminishes. If we are fortunate enough to keep all of our hair, graying hair can be a plus, adding an aura of experience and wisdom. But as our skin begins to wrinkle and sag, we are forced to face the reality of aging: Some things aren't going to be as good as they used to be.

A physical slowdown caused by the onset of aches and pains begins around middle age, but it is so gradual that we are not fully aware of the progressive and destructive effects of aging. With fewer worries and more time to travel and do the things we like to do, most of us enjoy life more than ever, despite the need to occasionally pop an aspirin or take a course of prescription medication. But there are some danger signs we should watch for, particularly when it comes to potentially disabling back and leg pain. We must be careful not to always attribute back pain to the aging process, especially when pain is persistent or appears suddenly without obvious cause. Back pain can reflect a variety of problems—some minor, some serious, and some potentially fatal. With these observations in mind, you owe it to yourself and your future to know something about what might be causing your back or leg pain and what you should do about it.

The Many Causes of Back and Leg Pain

Most commonly, back pain after middle age is caused by degenerative changes involving joints and intervertebral discs. As discs dehydrate with aging and become progressively thinner and fragmented, arthritic formations begin to build up around joints and vertebral bodies that begin to jam upon each other, causing chronic back trouble. Disc herniation is less common after age fifty because of a scarcity of disc cartilage. But spurs or osteophytes may begin to encroach upon the spinal canal (spinal stenosis) and upon the openings between the vertebrae where the spinal nerves exit (lateral stenosis). When one of these spurs touches or compresses a spinal nerve, radiation of pain into the lower leg (sciatica) may cause symptoms resembling disc herniation. In most cases, these symptoms will resolve with time, but the problem should be monitored by a physician who can check reflexes and measure muscle strength. If calf muscles begin to atrophy or shrink, or if weakness causes a foot drop (flopping your foot when you walk), an orthopedic specialist or a neurosurgeon should be consulted to consider surgery for removal of the spur or disc fragment. Utilizing such sophisticated diagnostic measures as magnetic resonance imaging (MRI), a physician can often pinpoint the problem and offer a definitive diagnosis.

Occasionally, thickened ligaments or bony overgrowth will encroach upon the spinal canal, causing pain and weakness in both legs while walking (neurogenic claudication). This can be a serious problem that might also require spinal surgery.

In rare cases, a disc herniation in the lower spine, usually at the L4 and L5 levels at the bottom of the spine, will protrude into the spinal canal and compress spinal nerves to cause sudden loss of control of the bladder and the bowels (cauda equina syndrome). The resulting urinary or fecal incontinence is a medical emergency that should immediately be brought to the attention of a neurosurgeon.

A "Horse's Tail" Problem

If you know that the words "cauda equina" are Latin for "horse's tail," you might be wondering why such a serious problem could have such a strange name. Here's why: The spinal cord ends at the level of the second lumbar vertebra, (remember, there are five lumbar vertebrae). Spinal nerves leaving the spinal cord hang down like the hair on a horse's tail and pass out between the lumbar vertebrae at lower levels to supply pelvic and leg structures. Nerves supplying pelvic structures pass through the solid bony structure of the sacrum at the very bottom of the spine (supporting the lumbar vertebrae) where there are no discs or joints to cause mischief. Just imagine what problems we would have—ranging from urinary incontinence to sexual impotence—if disc herniation and spur formation occurred in the sacrum. Thanks to nature's design, such problems are not common; when they do occur, they are usually the result of lumbar disc herniation, which can be surgically corrected.

What Is Causing Your Leg Pain?

Most of the time, pain radiating into the lower leg is a sciatic nerve pain caused by disc herniation or spur formation in the lower lumbar spine. But when there is pain and cramping in one or both legs after walking a block or two, there might be a circulatory problem. Typically, leg pain caused by circulatory insufficiency will consistently occur after walking a certain distance and then subside when you stop walking. The pain recurs when walking is resumed. Doctors call this peripheral vascular disease, or "intermittent claudication."

You might be referred to a vascular specialist if there is reason to believe that hardening of the arteries (arteriosclerosis) or some other problem, such as an aortic aneurysm or a tumor, is partially obstructing the flow of blood to your legs.

Sudden onset of severe and persistent leg pain that is accompanied by discoloration and decreased skin temperature may indicate an arterial blood clot. Without appropriate treatment, such a clot could lead to loss of a foot or leg. Pain, redness, tenderness, and swelling along the course of a vein may be caused by phlebitis, or inflammation of a vein. Clots that form in veins can break loose and travel to the lungs, a situation that can be life-threatening. *See a physician immediately if you develop sudden severe leg pain.* Let your doctor decide if your pain is the result of a blood clot or a sciatic nerve problem.

The Question of Cancer

Most of us are not concerned about a little stiffness or back pain that comes and goes. Generally, if you have Type M back pain caused by strain, arthritis, or some other muscle or joint problem, you feel pain only when you bend or move about. The pain can usually be relieved with rest, massage, and moist heat or a cold pack. But if you develop back pain that persists twenty-four hours a day and grows progressively worse day after day, unrelieved by treatment, you should begin to suspect that the pain might have an internal or organic origin. You should be especially concerned if the pain is not aggravated by bending and moving your body.

In my forty-three-year career as a chiropractor specializing in the care of back pain, I saw many patients who had back pain caused by cancer, a diseased organ, or some other problem unrelated to back and spinal structures. Many of these patients had a history of previously treated breast, lung, or prostate cancer. The cancer had recurred or spread to another site, causing referred back pain. Sometimes, the cancer will spread to the ribs or the vertebrae, eating away the inside of the bone so that no pain is felt on movement until the disease is far advanced. This is why physicians should always examine the site of the pain before deciding that the pain is referred from somewhere else.

In some cases, referred back pain occurs long before the cancer is discovered in a remote part of the body. I remember seeing a pharmacist, for example, who visited my office complaining of shoulder and upper back pain. He had spent many months treating himself with medication to relieve the pain. When I examined him, his musculoskeletal structures were normal. Jarring, probing, and movement would not elicit pain. A chest X ray revealed a malignant tumor in the upper lobe of his lung on the side of the shoulder pain.

Remember: If you develop persistent, progressive pain that is unrelieved by rest and not aggravated by movement, see your doctor as soon as possible.

What about Kidney Stones?

A stone passing from the kidney to the bladder (through the ureter) can cause severe back and groin pain that may be accompanied by muscle spasm, nausea, and other symptoms. Unlike Type M back pain that is relieved by rest, the pain of a kidney stone causes restless movement that forces you to seek relief from pain by constantly changing positions, even when you are doubled over in agony. When one of my patients called my office to tell me that his back was "out of place," I advised him to go to a hospital emergency room when he told me that he was literally rolling around on the floor. They found a kidney stone lodged in his ureter.

A constant backache without pain on movement but accompanied by fever may be the result of a kidney or prostate infection. You should always take your temperature when you have unrelenting backache or a urinary problem.

You don't have to be a doctor to figure out that if you are pacing the floor with severe back pain, it's not likely that your back is at fault.

Osteoporosis as a Cause of Back Pain

Unfortunately, as we age, many of us become less active. We might also skimp on meals, underestimating the importance of a good diet. Some of us might be taking corticosteroids to stem or relieve arthritic inflammation. All of these factors can contribute to the development of bone-weakening osteoporosis, a disease affecting twenty-five million Americans. It occurs six times more often in women than in men.

When osteoporosis is advanced, it can result in collapse (or crush fracture) of brittle and porous vertebrae. This happens most often in post-menopausal women who may develop calcium-deficient bones when their estrogen level drops at menopause. One out of three women has osteoporosis! The disease also occurs in men, but usually at a later age than in women—after age sixty-five, for example. It's important for both men and women to make sure that their diets supply adequate calcium and vitamin D to help *prevent* osteoporosis in the early years of life—long before the age the disease is expected to appear. Even though bone loss may begin after age thirty, osteoporosis may not show up on a plain X-ray exam until bones have lost up to 40 percent of their mineral content. Sudden appearance of a "dowager's hump" in a painful back, or gradual development of a hump after menopause, may signal collapse of one or more mineral deficient vertebrae. Many cases of spontaneous hip fracture have occurred before the stricken individuals even knew that they had osteoporosis.

Remember that calcium requirement increases as you grow older. Adults under the age of fifty need 1,000 milligrams of calcium daily. Post-menopausal women and everyone over the age of sixty-five need 1,500 milligrams of calcium daily. The older you become, the more important it is to eat low-fat, calcium-rich foods. When there is doubt about your calcium intake, take a calcium supplement.

Osteoporosis can be detected early by undergoing bone mineral density testing with an X-ray densitometer. When appropriate, a physician can prescribe hormone replacement therapy or a bone-building drug such as alendronate (Fosamax) or calcitonin (a hormone) to halt destruction of bone.

For more on osteoporosis and your back, see Chapter 4.

Exercise Is Important

Even if your diet is good and you are getting adequate calcium, vitamin D, and other micronutrients needed to build strong bones, your bones will remain only as strong as they need to be to withstand the amount of stress placed upon them. This is why it is so important to stay active and get plenty of exercise, no matter how old you might be. Staying strong and healthy tends to prolong an active sex life, which in itself is a form of exercise that stimulates production of hormones needed to look younger and live longer.

Even when you hurt your back, you should not remain inactive for very long. Bed rest should be limited to three of four days. Prolonged rest or inactivity weakens bones and muscles and may contribute to the formation of blood clots. Try to resume your exercise program as soon as possible when you are recovering from injury or illness. When you need medication to relieve pain and stiffness, first try taking aspirin, acetaminophen (Tylenol), or some nonsteroidal over-the-counter anti-inflammatory product. Such medications should be used sparingly, however. Too much aspirin (acetyl-salicylic acid) can inflame your stomach, while high doses of acetamino-phen can damage your liver. If you are taking a blood thinner or some other prescription medication, you should not take any medication without your doctor's permission.

If you must resort to opioids and other prescription drugs to relieve back pain, you may not be ready for any exercise other than simple walk-ing. Always check with your physician. If you have gout, rheumatoid arthri-tis, or some other serious inflammatory disease causing back pain, your doctor may have to prescribe special medication and place limitations on the amount and type of exercise you do.

Follow these basic rules:

1. Stay physically active and exercise regularly.

2. Eat a variety of fresh, natural foods every day, including low-fat, calcium-rich foods.

3. Enjoy life with a happy, optimistic outlook.

Watch for these red flags:

1. Back pain that occurs after a fall or an injury should always be brought to the attention of a physician, especially if you are taking corticosteroids or if you have a history of cancer.

2. Persistent back pain that is unrelieved by rest, not aggravated by movement, or is associated with fever or unexplained weight loss warrants immediate medical attention.

3. When there is sudden onset of severe leg pain that persists unrelieved, blood clots should be ruled out before making a diagnosis of sciatica.

SUMMARY

1. Intervertebral disc cartilage tends to dehydrate and degenerate as we grow older, making disc herniation less common after age fifty.

2. When leg pain occurs, it's always important to distinguish nerve pain from a possibly more serious vascular problem.

3. Sciatic nerve pain commonly affects only a portion of the leg below the knee and may weaken calf and foot muscles.

4. Sudden onset of severe pain affecting the entire leg could be a sign of a dangerous arterial blood clot.

5. Leg pain that recurs consistently after walking a certain distance may be a vascular insufficiency caused by hardening of the arteries, or arteriosclerosis.

6. Back pain aggravated by movement and relieved by rest is usually mechanical in origin.

7. Persistent back pain unrelieved by rest or treatment and not aggravated by movement may be referred pain that has an internal origin.

8. Sudden loss of control of bladder and bowels could be caused by a tumor or by a protrusion of a herniated disc into the spinal canal.

9. Sudden or gradual appearance of a spinal hump after middle age may indicate collapse of osteoporotic vertebrae.

10. It's important to exercise regularly and eat properly to strengthen bones and muscles and to keep blood vessels open.

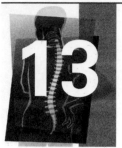

When You Need the Help of a Specialist

No matter what type of back trouble you think you have, it's usually best to consult with your family physician before seeking specialized medical care. If your health insurance is controlled by managed care or a health maintenance organization (HMO), you may be *forced* to see an authorized general physician before you can see any kind of specialist. Increasing numbers of employers and insurance carriers are switching to managed care in the interest of efficiency and reduced costs. Your primary care physician will decide what type of care you need and then refer you to the appropriate specialist—if needed.

There are many causes of back pain, some of which do not originate in the back. A general practitioner can usually recognize mechanical (Type M) back pain as opposed to symptoms felt in the back but caused by kidney trouble, a stomach ulcer, a diseased gall bladder, pancreatic cancer, an aneurysm, or some other organic (Type O) problem.

Your family physician, who is familiar with your body and your history, can very often predict or anticipate the development of symptoms, allowing him or her to begin proper treatment without delay. Or your doctor might refer you to a specialist. If your back pain is caused by something inside your body (Type O), you might be referred to an internist. Type M back troubles might be referred to an orthopedist. Symptoms involving the nervous system might best be handled by a neurologist or a neurosurgeon. Progressive arthritis, especially in young people, should always be brought to the attention of a rheumatologist, a physician who specializes in the treatment of arthritis.

As a lay person, it might not be wise for you to bypass your family physician and attempt to decide for yourself what kind of a specialist you should see for a diagnosis of your back pain. Going to the wrong specialist can be a frustrating, expensive experience, not to mention the delay it can cause in getting early and appropriate treatment for your problem. Furthermore, some diagnostic and treatment procedures, when not indicated, might be harmful to your body, as in the case of a CAT scan or a cortisone injection. It's therefore always a good idea to have a trustworthy family physician who can screen your symptoms and guide your selection of a specialist in caring for your health, including back trouble.

Mechanical conditions involving the back and spine can often be handled effectively by a chiropractor. There are, in fact, certain types of back trouble that are best treated with spinal manipulation, which is the chiropractor's forte.

Manipulation can also be performed by an osteopath or a physiatrist (a physician specializing in physical medicine) A few orthopedic specialists now perform manipulation as well. Some physical therapists also manipulate or mobilize the spine, though not as extensively as a chiropractor, whose primary method of treatment is manipulating the spinal joints. Orthopedic specialists often refer patients to chiropractors who use spinal manipulation in a scientific, selective manner, especially when there is evidence that spinal joints are not moving properly.

Obviously, no one doctor can diagnose and treat every condition that affects your back. Without the correct diagnosis, it's impossible to determine what type of doctor you need. Anytime you have back symptoms that persist longer than four weeks, get a second opinion if there is any doubt about the diagnosis.

Specialists in a Nutshell

■ **Internal medicine and family practice physicians** are primary care physicians who can diagnose and treat most ailments and are able to detect problems that might need specialized care. Patients with back pain that persists unrelieved for several weeks may be referred to the appropriate specialist by a primary care doctor, depending upon the diagnosis.

■ A **physiatrist,** a physician who specializes in nonsurgical treatment of musculoskeletal problems, is often the best doctor to see for persistent Type M back pain.

■ An **orthopedic surgeon** may be needed if there is evidence of disease or damaging injury to musculoskeletal structures, as in the case of arthritis, fractures, or torn muscles or ligaments. Some orthopedists specialize in spinal treatment.

■ A **neurologist** specializes in diagnosis and treatment of nonsurgical conditions that have symptoms involving the nervous system. A neurologist is less likely to recommend surgery than a neurosurgeon, who does nothing but surgery. So it's sometimes a good idea to see a neurologist before seeing a neurosurgeon when there is arm or leg pain associated with back pain.

■ A **neurosurgeon** specializes in the use of surgery needed to correct problems involving the brain, spinal cord, or spinal nerves, as in the case of brain tumors, disc herniations, and other conditions that may damage the nervous system.

■ An **osteopath,** who generally combines traditional medical care with manipulative procedures, can manage a variety of Type M problems involving muscles and joints.

■ A **chiropractor,** who specializes in the care of Type M neuromusculoskeletal problems and hands-on spinal manipulation, can often relieve neck and back pain and related problems by loosening stiff or impaired spinal joints.

■ A **physical therapist** specializes in the use of a variety of physical treatment methods to restore or improve physical functions.

The Specialty of Family Practice

The practice of medicine has become so complicated and vast in its scope that many medical specialties have been developed to utilize numerous and new methods of diagnosing and treating disease. The job of a family physician, who must recognize an ailment in order to treat it or refer you to the appropriate specialist, is becoming increasingly complex. For this reason, family practice, like internal medicine, is now a medical specialty requiring two additional years of training after acquiring an M.D. degree. (It usually takes nine years to earn a medical degree—four years of college, four years of medical school, and one year of internship in a hospital.)

COMMON PHYSICAL TREATMENT MODALITIES IN BRIEF

- **Acupuncture.** A controversial method of puncturing the skin with needles for pain relief that may be the result of a placebo effect or the release of endorphins in the brain.

- **Chiropractic.** Use of "spinal adjustments" to correct "subluxations" as a method of "restoring and maintaining health" and treating back pain.

- **Cold pack.** Use of cold to ease pain, restrict blood flow, and reduce swelling or inflammation in muscles and joints.

- **Counter irritation.** Use of liniments to produce skin irritation in order to diminish perception of pain.

- **Diathermy.** A short wave frequency applied over a body part to stimulate blood flow and healing by generating heat deep within the tissues.

- **Electrical stimulation.** Use of an electric current to tone muscles, pump out waste products, stimulate healing, and ease pain.

- **Hot pack.** Moist heat applied to increase blood flow, ease pain, and relax muscles.

- **Hydrotherapy.** Use of water in baths, whirlpools, packs, compresses, and other ways to apply hot or cold water for therapeutic purposes.

- **Manipulation.** Manual movement of joints to restore mobility, often used by chiropractors and osteopaths.

- **Massage.** Kneading and rubbing muscles to stimulate blood flow, relax muscles, and improve the function of muscles and joints.

- **Physical therapy.** Use of a variety of physical treatment methods for relieving pain and improving or restoring physical ability.

- **Rehabilitation.** Use of exercise and other physical treatment methods to aid recovery from physical disability caused by disease or injury.

- **Transcutaneous electrical stimulation (TENS).** Use of a small battery-powered device connected to electrodes placed over a painful area to modify pain perception.

- **Traction.** Stretching the spine to relieve muscle spasm and pressure on joints, discs, and spinal nerves.

- **Ultrasound.** High-frequency sound waves used to generate heat below the skin's surface, breaking up tissue deposits and reducing congestion.

With increasing emphasis on managed care, today's family practitioner is becoming more concerned about prevention and health maintenance. If you're fortunate enough to have a certified family practice specialist as your family physician, you may have the best of starting points for caring for all your ailments, including back problems.

Orthopedists and Neurosurgeons

An orthopedist may be the first specialist your family physician will refer you to for diagnosis and treatment of a severe or persistent back problem. With five additional years of training after medical school, orthopedic specialists know more about the musculoskeletal structures than any other practitioner. They are especially adept at surgical repair of damaged muscles, joints, ligaments, and bones. Diagnosis and treatment of back trouble is only a part of the practice of orthopedics, although a few orthopedists do specialize in back and spinal care. Some specialize in sports medicine.

Very often, an orthopedic specialist will refer patients to a physical therapist for treatment of a diagnosed problem. He might also refer selected patients to a chiropractor or osteopath for manipulation.

When back or neck pain involves the nervous system, your doctor might refer you to a neurologist or neurosurgeon. Diseases of the nervous system are best diagnosed by a neurologist. But if you need surgery for a condition involving the brain, spinal cord, or spinal nerves, a neurosurgeon is the perfect person for the job. Treatment of spinal conditions such as disc herniation or spinal stenosis, when they involve the spinal cord or the spinal nerves, may also require the attention of a neurosurgeon.

Like orthopedic surgeons, neurosurgeons must have five additional years of training after medical school in order to be certified in their specialty.

Physiatrists and Rehabilitation

Physiatrists, or specialists in physical medicine, are concerned primarily with diseases and disorders of the neuromuscular system (function of nerves and muscles). The treatment given by physiatrists includes the use of all physical measures needed to aid recovery from disease or injury and to speed recovery of physical ability.

After completion of medical school, a physiatrist must have three years of additional training followed by two years of specialty practice before taking board examinations.

Physiatrists often include the use of manipulation in their treatment armamentarium. Since there are so few physiatrists in private practice, manipulation is more immediately available from a chiropractor or an osteopath, however.

Internists: The Diagnosticians

A specialist in internal medicine is often of great help in determining the origin of back pain referred from an internal source, as from the gall bladder or the pancreas. As the ultimate diagnostician, an internist can often diagnose and treat a variety of organic and systemic diseases.

A general internist must complete two years of residency in internal medicine after medical school. If an internist has a subspecialty such as cardiology, gastroenterology, or endocrinology, he or she has completed two additional years of training.

Radiology: X-ray Specialists

Most doctors depend upon radiologists to take and interpret X rays for diagnosis of bone and soft tissue problems. With new advances in computerized tomography (CAT scan), magnetic resonance imaging (MRI), contrast imaging, and other high-tech imaging procedures, it takes a radiologist to interpret the films produced by such testing.

A diagnostic radiologist must complete a four-year residency after medical school to be board certified. Subspecialties in radiology, such as neuroradiology (imaging of the nervous system) or uroradiology (imaging of the urinary tract), may require additional fellowship in radiology.

Rheumatologists: The Arthritis Doctors

Arthritis, gout, lupus erythematosus, fibromyalgia, and other diseases that inflame muscles and destroy joints are so common and complicated that a specialist called a rheumatologist is required for diagnosis and treatment of these diseases.

A rheumatologist is an internist who has completed two or more additional years of training in rheumatology.

Osteopaths: Diversified Doctors

Doctors of osteopathy (D.O.s), who employ manipulation along with medical procedures, have educational requirements almost identical to those of medical doctors (M.D.s). Osteopathy offers general practice as well as specialty and subspecialty practices.

Although some osteopaths abandon the use of manipulation in their practice, back patients often seek the services of an osteopath (usually a general practitioner) who can prescribe medication as well as perform manipulation.

Chiropractors as Back Specialists

Most of us think of a doctor of chiropractic (D.C.) as a back specialist. When we need spinal manipulation, it will probably be done by a chiropractor, since 94 percent of all spinal manipulation performed in the United States is done by chiropractors. Few chiropractors claim to be back specialists, however. In keeping with the fundamental chiropractic theory that spinal manipulation can restore and maintain health by removing nerve interference in the vertebral column, many chiropractors claim to have effective treatments for a variety of organic ailments as well as back pain.

It's not uncommon these days for a physician to refer a back-pain patient to a properly limited chiropractor for spinal manipulation. If the chiropractor offers a treatment for organic disease or attempts to use a mallet to tap vertebrae into alignment (see page 265), my advice would be to find another chiropractor who specializes in the care of neck and back pain and other neuromusculoskeletal problems and who performs manual manipulation.

In the fall of 2001, the minimum undergraduate admission requirement at United States chiropractic colleges increased from two years to three years. Some chiropractic colleges will soon require a baccalaureate for admission. A few states (about four at this time) require a preprofessional baccalaureate for licensure. Chiropractic college requires four years.

Chiropractors do not prescribe drugs or perform surgery. While most chiropractors use physical therapy along with manipulation, a few chiropractic colleges teach "straight chiropractic," which maintains that vertebral subluxation (misalignment) is the major cause of disease and that spinal manipulation is the only treatment needed. There is no evidence, however, that subluxations cause disease or that spinal adjustments can cure any disease.

Since chiropractic is a limited treatment method, one that employs manipulation and other physical treatment modalities, chiropractors are necessarily limited practitioners who function best in the care of Type M neck and back pain and other neuromusculoskeletal problems. Any chiropractors who specialize in pediatrics and similar fields cannot be taken seriously.

Children should be treated by pediatricians and not by chiropractors who often attempt to treat ear infections, colic, and similar ailments, most of which are self-limiting but potentially serious. Backache is rare in small children; when it does occur, it could be an indication of a serious organic problem and should always be brought to the attention of a pediatrician.

THE MIND/BODY CONNECTION

There is evidence to indicate that the mind has much to do with the amount of pain you feel. Negative thoughts and depression, for example, can open the "pain gate" in your spinal cord, while a good state of mind with positive thoughts can close it. Doctors call this the "gate control theory." This may explain, in part, why people who are optimistic about a treatment method will often feel less pain and recover more rapidly than a person who does not believe in a treatment method. This is one reason some ineffective remedies can actually result in improvement or cure through a placebo effect. Fear and negative thoughts, on the other hand, can result in illness through a nocebo effect (a bad effect that is the opposite of a good placebo effect).

Emotional stress has been labeled a cause of "tension myositis syndrome," a form of back pain that can be cured only by a relaxed and positive state of mind. Apparently, a mind/body connection can be used to ease pain and speed healing or it can cause or increase pain and suffering, causing psychosomatic illnesses such as headaches, backaches, gastrointestinal symptoms, and so on. You should always make sure that your illness has been correctly diagnosed in order to determine if you have a disease or organic illness that requires a specific treatment. Then, no matter what type of illness you have, a positive, relaxed, and optimistic state of mind can be used to enhance the type of treatment you receive.

The back problems of pre-teen children are rarely like those of adults who may have degenerative changes and other problems that stiffen the spine. The spine of an infant or a child under the age of ten or twelve has cartilaginous (soft) growth centers and may have undetected spinal abnormalities that could be damaged by spinal manipulation. There are few, if any, indications of a need for spinal manipulation in the treatment of a small child.

It is not a good idea to subject a child to the radiation of an X-ray examination unless there is persistent mechanical-type pain or a history of injury, which should be evaluated by a pediatrician or an orthopedist. It's never a good idea to take a child to a chiropractor when there is fever or infection. There is no justification for X-raying children so that their spines can be manipulated as a treatment for disease or infection—as done by many "chiropractic pediatricians." Simply put, a chiropractor is not a pediatrician and should not be treating a small child unless referred by an orthopedist for a special reason.

So while spinal manipulation can be effective in the treatment of certain types of neck and back pain and related problems (such as tension headache and arm or leg pain), you must be as cautious in your selection of a chiropractor as your chiropractor should be in accepting you as a patient. With more and more chiropractors specializing in the care of neuromusculoskeletal problems, it is becoming increasingly likely that your family physician or an HMO will refer you to a chiropractor for care of your back pain. A drugless practitioner who can treat Type M aches and pains with manipulation and physical therapy is often a good choice when he is integrated into a health-care system in which doctors in all fields work together.

Physical Therapists and Body Care

A physical therapist uses physical treatment methods, often including use of manipulation, to relieve pain, restore function, improve mobility, and prevent or limit permanent physical disabilities in patients suffering from injuries or disease.

As of 2002, accredited physical therapy programs were required to offer a master's degree; some even offer a doctoral degree.

Last-Resort Surgical Remedies for Back Problems

Only about 1 percent of all spine surgeries are emergencies that dictate the need for surgery and require quick action. In 99 percent of cases, spinal surgery is elective, which means that it is a choice you must make. When conservative treatment methods fail and you do not feel that you can live with your back problem, a surgical procedure might be considered. Here are some of the most common back surgeries done by orthopedists and neurosurgeons:

■ **Chemonucleosis** (chymopapain injection) involves injection of an enzyme into a herniated disc to dissolve the gelatinous portion of the disc protrusion. Since there is a risk of infection, allergic reaction, and paralysis, this procedure is not often done in the United States.

■ **Percutaneous discectomy** uses a laser or suction device, inserted through a small incision, to remove a portion of a herniated disc.

■ **Microsurgical discectomy** is performed through an incision less than one inch long. It's used primarily to remove the portion of a disc herniation that is compressing a nerve root.

■ **Laminectomy** requires removal of a portion of the back of a vertebra to permit removal of a bony growth or herniated disc that might be encroaching on the spinal canal or upon spinal nerves.

■ **Spinal fusion** is used to prevent movement between two trouble-making vertebrae. Bone grafts or metallic fixation devices may be used to hold the vertebrae together or to allow them to grow (fuse) together.

Note: Remember that any kind of spinal surgery is not to be taken lightly. A specific need for surgery must be demonstrated, and it should be done only if absolutely necessary. When surgery is really needed, dramatic relief of symptoms should occur. But when surgery is unnecessary or done for the wrong reasons, symptoms may persist or worsen, resulting in "failed back surgery syndrome" (back or leg pain that continues after spinal surgery).

Surgery can sometimes be avoided by using spinal epidural steroid injections, in which a steroid or anesthetic is injected into spinal canal membranes surrounding a painful disc or spinal nerve. This may relieve pain and inflammation enough to allow natural healing to occur. Facet injections may be used when it is believed that pain is originating in spinal joints.

SUMMARY

1. The office of a trusted family physician is usually the best starting place for guidance in the care of back pain.

2. The services of a specialist in internal medicine are sometimes needed to determine the source of back pain referred from inside the body.

3. Diseased or damaged muscles, joints, ligaments, and bones, especially those needing surgical repair, are best handled by an orthopedic surgeon.

4. A neurologist, who does not perform surgery, is trained to diagnose symptoms involving the nervous system.

5. Back surgery for conditions affecting the spinal cord or the spinal nerves may best be performed by a neurosurgeon.

6. Rehabilitation of persons disabled by injury or surgery may need the long-range care of a physiatrist, a physician who specializes in physical medicine.

7. An osteopath, a practitioner who combines conventional medical care with spinal manipulation and other physical treatment methods, can often handle back problems effectively.

8. Chiropractors, whose methods of treatment are limited to manipulation and physical therapy, are perhaps most skillful in the use of spinal manipulation.

9. Although spinal manipulation is an effective treatment for certain types of neck and back trouble and related problems, there is no evidence that it is effective in the treatment and prevention of organic disease.

10. If back pain persists or grows worse after four weeks, get a second opinion to make sure that your problem has been correctly diagnosed.

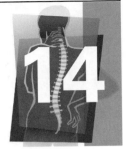

Sense and Nonsense in Chiropractic Care of Back Pain

Chiropractors are gaining acceptance in the mainstream of health care as neuromusculoskeletal specialists. While there is much a good chiropractor can do to help you with tension headache and a variety of Type M aches and pains, not all chiropractors are alike, and their treatment methods may vary. You may have to shop around to find a chiropractor who has the right treatment method and a properly limited practice.

Basically, there are two types of chiropractors. One type treats only with adjustments or spinal manipulation, and one type uses physical therapy along with manipulation. The type of chiropractor who treats only with spinal adjustments is known as a "straight" or "subluxation-based" chiropractor and may offer treatment for the broad scope of human (and sometimes animal) ailments. A chiropractor who uses physical therapy along with spinal manipulation, also called a "mixer" chiropractor, tends to be more conservative in the scope of his or her practice.

The reason for this difference in chiropractors is that the original chiropractic theory, supported by straight chiropractors, maintains that vertebral misalignment, or subluxation, causes most diseases and that spinal adjustment is the only treatment needed for any ailment. The mixer chiropractor, who does not totally adhere to this theory, may include other treatment methods and may be less inclined to use spinal manipulation as a treatment for organic disease. With a greater variety of treatment methods, a mixer chiropractor may have more to offer in relieving the symptoms of back pain. But remember that both straight and mixer chiropractors may attempt to treat organic disease by adjusting "vertebral subluxations." And a mixer chiropractor may include use of such unproven "alternative" remedies as homeopathy, herbology, colonic irrigation, megavitamins, or chelation therapy. So when you do find a chiropractor who can relieve your back pain, that does not mean that you should allow the chiropractor to treat your disease and infections, no matter what kind of chiropractor or what type of treatment.

Whenever possible, it's always best to seek the services of a chiropractor who limits his or her practice to the care of neck and back pain and other Type M problems and who uses both physical therapy and hands-on manipulation. This type of chiropractor works better with medical practitioners, is generally more recognized in the scientific community, and is usually preferred by managed-care organizations.

Finding a Chiropractic Back Specialist [5]

The case of Susan B. is a good example of the difficulty that a back patient might have finding a properly limited chiropractor.

Over a period of a couple of years, Susan visited my office several times for treatment of muscle spasm caused by irritation in a deformed and arthritic joint in her lower spine. Each time she came, all she needed was a little gentle spinal manipulation along with ultrasound, electrical stimulation, or some other form of physical therapy. After only a few treatments, she would get along fine for several months—until she reinjured her back. She would then call for another appointment.

A few months after Susan's last visit to my office, she moved to another state. When she hurt her back moving furniture, she went to a local chiropractor. That night, she called my home, obviously distressed and frightened.

"Doctor Homola," Susan began with a note of restrained urgency, "I went to a chiropractor today to get treatment for my lower back. He made X rays of my neck and my back and told me they were both out of alignment and that it would take thirty-eight treatments to straighten me out. He said that if I did not complete the full course of treatments, my spine might degenerate and my health would deteriorate. Is that possible? He wants me to pay for the treatments in advance so that I can get a discount, and he wants $3,000. What should I do?"

Needless to say, I advised Susan not to go back to that chiropractor. I offered her a few guidelines to follow in finding another chiropractor—one who would treat her back trouble without any associated nonsense.

How to Avoid Questionable Chiropractors

Here is what I tell people who are looking for an ethical and properly limited chiropractor:

Beware of Unneessary X-ray Exams and the Inappropriate Use of Thermography

Do not respond to chiropractic advertisements that offer free exams, especially X rays or thermography! Exposure to unnecessary radiation with an X-ray machine may be harmful to your body. "Free" X rays or thermography may lead to more X rays, resulting in additional radiation as well as unexpected expense.

Not everyone needs an X-ray exam. Generally, if you don't have a history of disease or injury, and your back pain occurs following simple exertion or a stumble, chances are it will resolve in a few days or after a few weeks. A little time and observation are often all that is needed to diagnose and treat a simple back strain or a neck spasm. X-ray exam is often not indicated in the case of nonspecific back pain unless symptoms persist longer than four weeks.

"Straight" chiropractors, who maintain that vertebral subluxation is a cause of disease, often X-ray the spine repeatedly in order to adjust specific vertebrae as a preventive measure. Such chiropractors might recommend treatment for infants and children as well as for adults. The result is that some chiropractors might be using X rays unnecessarily to adjust imaginary or harmless vertebral misalignments. This might be a waste of time and money as well as a danger to health, especially in the case of infants and children. When simple lower back pain is present, X rays are generally recommended only when symptoms have been present for longer than a month or when there are certain red flags indicating disease (such as osteoporosis or cancer) or serious injury. You do not need an X-ray exam when you have no symptoms or when it is used in a search for "subluxations" labeled as a cause of disease or infection.

Thermography, a method of photographing color caused by heat changes in the skin, has limited diagnostic value and is often offered free to attract new patients. These patients may then be advised to submit to X-ray examination based on the color patterns demonstrated on thermography prints.

In comparing thermography color patterns on both sides of the body, government investigators found that thermograms were often interpreted as abnormal in normal, healthy persons (Agency for Healthcare Research and Quality, publication No. 95–0642). Colorful thermography prints are a great gimmick for promoting further examination with X rays.

Some chiropractors use questionable heat-detecting instruments to locate "subluxations" prior to spinal adjustment.

Don't Worry about the Alignment of Your Vertebrae

Don't be overly concerned that you might have misaligned vertebrae that might be surreptitiously damaging your health. If you do not have any pain and you can move around normally, it's not likely that you have a vertebra out of place that needs correction by manipulation.

Many of us have chronic vertebral misalignments that are the result of spinal curvatures, joint abnormalities, disc degeneration, and other common mechanical problems. While these misalignments might cause some Type M back pain, they are often insignificant and usually not correctable. When pain and spasm do occur, spinal manipulation will often relieve symptoms by restoring mobility in the affected joints.

When you do undergo spinal manipulation, you might hear and feel your vertebral joints pop, or crack. This does not mean, however, that your vertebrae are out of place. While a binding spinal joint might pop when mobility is restored, normal joints will also pop. Chiropractic patients who believe that their vertebrae pop because they are out of place often feel that they need regular manipulation to keep their vertebrae in proper alignment. If the chiropractor performing the manipulation recommends regular treatment in a preventive maintenance program, the patient might become psychologically addicted to spine-popping manipulation. Unfortunately, some chiropractors believe that vertebral misalignment can cause disease and that regular spinal adjustments are needed to restore and maintain health. It's not unusual for some chiropractors to adjust the spine as a treatment for allergies, ear infections, or stomach trouble. Some claim to be able to prevent colds, flu, and other common infections by manipulating the spine to boost the body's immune system. There is no evidence to support such treatment.

A "Pinched Nerve" Will Not Affect Your General Health

Spinal nerves are commonly irritated or pinched by herniated discs, bony spurs, and other degenerative changes in the spine. When this happens, there may be pain, numbness, tingling, and other symptoms radiating into musculoskeletal structures supplied by the affected nerves, usually in one arm or one leg. So it's not likely that you would have a pinched nerve without being aware of these symptoms.

Fortunately, spinal nerves primarily supply musculoskeletal structures. With the exception of muscles controlling the bladder and the bowels, spinal nerves do not have controlling influence over the function of internal

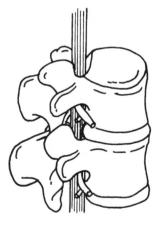

Figure 14-1. There is normally plenty of room between vertebrae for the passage of spinal nerves. Pinching of a nerve occurs only when there is disc herniation, spur formation, thickening of ligaments or cartilage, or some other pathological process.

organs. When a spinal nerve is damaged, there may be weakness and shrinkage in the muscles supplied by the nerve. There may also be loss of sensation in the skin over the affected muscles. But there is no evidence to indicate that pinching or even cutting a spinal nerve will affect organic function. Even when the back is broken, shutting off the flow of nerve impulses through the spinal nerves, the internal organs continue to function, even though the victim's arms and legs may be paralyzed. The reason for this is that the internal organs are supplied primarily by a separate autonomic nervous system that does not depend upon one spinal nerve to function.

If a fracture or dislocation involves any of the top four vertebrae in the neck, damage to the brain stem can cause respiratory failure or death.

Severance of the spinal cord in the lower portion of the cervical spine can cause quadriplegia, or paralysis in both arms and both legs. Crushing or cutting of the spinal cord near the waist can cause paraplegia, or loss of use of both legs. In either case, the injury is not fatal.

If a chiropractor tells you that you have a pinched spinal nerve that might affect your general health or that you need regular spinal adjustments to prevent disease caused by "nerve interference," be suspicious. If you do develop symptoms of a pinched nerve, you can be fairly certain that the symptoms are the result of a herniated disc or a degenerative condition and not the result of a slightly misaligned vertebra.

When you have arm or leg pain that is worsened by treatment with manipulation, discontinue the treatment and seek the opinion of a neurologist or a neurosurgeon.

Warning: It's important to remember that since spinal nerves supply musculoskeletal structures, they also supply some of the sphincter muscles involved in voluntary control of the bladder and the anal area. If a disc herniated into your spinal canal, there may be pressure on spinal nerves that travel down and pass through the solid, jointless sacrum at the bottom of your spine to supply bladder and anal muscles. Sudden loss of bladder or bowel control while you are having back pain presents a medical emergency that requires the immediate attention of a neurosurgeon.

Don't Pay for Chiropractic Treatments in Advance

A few chiropractors ask their patients to pay for long courses of treatments in advance. They may attempt to justify this by saying that it is in the best interest of the patient to complete the recommended number of treatments and that the patient can best be persuaded to do so by receiving a discount on prepaid treatments. Treatment may then be continued on a "preventive maintenance" basis.

Actually, it is difficult or impossible to determine beforehand how many treatments a patient might need. Sometimes, neck or back pain will be relieved with one or two treatments, making further treatment unnecessary. Simple back strain usually resolves in less than two weeks. A neck crick, which some of us occasionally wake up with, may disappear in four or five days.

I usually advise my patients to go by the way they feel and to discontinue treatment when they feel better. If treatment aggravates their pain, or if symptoms have not subsided after a couple of weeks, a different treatment or a different doctor might be indicated. It would be unwise to pay for a long course of treatments in advance if there is a chance that you need only a few treatments or if there is a question about the need for such treatment.

I do not recommend continued chiropractic manipulation when there are no obvious symptoms. Routine, ceremonial manipulation of a normal, healthy spine in an asymptomatic patient for preventive maintenance may be a waste of time and money, as well as a potential cause of injury. Chronic back pain caused by arthritis, disc degeneration, spinal curvature, or some other mechanical problem might be relieved by occasional spinal manipulation. But remember that popping your vertebrae with frequent manipulation in a preventive maintenance program will not prevent disease or maintain health. My advice is to get spinal manipulation when you need it and when you feel it helps and to avoid such treatment when you are not having symptoms related to neck or back trouble.

Adjusting Machines Are Not an Adequate Substitute for Manual Manipulation

Some chiropractors who feel that a slight misalignment of a vertebra is harmful to health may use a spring-loaded mallet to tap vertebrae "back into place." Vertebral misalignment most often occurs as a result of structural or degenerative changes in the spine. When a vertebra is freely movable, however, its alignment cannot be changed. If there is loss of mobility in a vertebral joint because of adhesions, binding, overriding joint surfaces, or muscle spasm, spinal manipulation performed by hand is the treatment of choice for restoration of mobility. Only a few treatments would be needed to unlock a joint.

Manipulation Is Best Combined with Physical Therapy

There are many causes of back pain, requiring many different types of treatment. Spinal manipulation is only one treatment among many and is not always indicated in the treatment of a neck or back problem. Physical therapy modalities, such as ultrasound, electrical stimulation, or diathermy, are often useful alone or in combination with spinal manipulation, especially in the case of muscular or ligamentous injuries. For this reason, I always advise my patients to find a chiropractor who uses physical treatment methods as well as manipulation in his or her office.

Doctors Must Work Together

No one doctor can always have the right treatment for your neck or back pain. Since chiropractors are drugless practitioners, they cannot offer you the medication you might need for a painful injury. Also, certain medical diagnostic methods are not available in chiropractors' offices. It may often be necessary to see a medical practitioner for diagnosis and treatment of an acutely painful or protracted back problem. A good chiropractor will not hesitate to refer you to the appropriate medical specialist when necessary. Conversely, if your chiropractor has a good reputation and a properly limited practice, your medical doctor will not discourage you from seeing him or her when you need spinal manipulation.

Note: The opinions expressed in this chapter are the author's and do not represent that of any chiropractic association or organization. Additional information about controversial chiropractic treatment based on vertebral subluxation theory can be found online at www.chirobase.org and www.chiromed.org.

SUMMARY

1. A properly limited chiropractor can offer an effective treatment for certain types of neck and back problems and related symptoms, such as tension headache and arm or leg pain.

2. As a chiropractor, I do not personally recommend chiropractic manipulation as a treatment for disease and infection.

3. I advise my patients to avoid chiropractors who advertise free X-ray or thermography exams.

4. I recommend chiropractors who specialize in the care of neuromusculoskeletol problems and who use both manipulation and physical therapy in their practice.

5. It is my opinion that spinal manipulation should be done by hand and not by adjusting machines or with mallets.

6. When you have severe back or leg pain and the diagnosis is in doubt, see an orthopedic specialist or a neurologist for another opinion.

7. "Straight" chiropractors, who use only spinal adjustment as a treatment, may not have as much to offer for back pain as a "mixer" chiropractor, who includes other treatment methods.

8. I do not recommend chiropractic treatment for newborn babies and infants!

9. If back pain has not improved after two to four weeks of treatment, discontinue the treatment and seek another opinion.

10. Spinal manipulation may be discontinued when symptoms are no longer present.

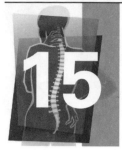

15

Questions Patients Commonly Ask about Back Trouble

Just about everything you need to know about how to care for your back in a self-help program is covered in this book. There are, however, always a few questions left unanswered. This final chapter will be devoted entirely to questions I commonly hear in my office. Perhaps it will answer a few of your questions.

 What causes the bump at the bottom of my neck where my neck and shoulders come together?

 The last vertebra at the bottom of the cervical spine normally has a long spinous process that projects out much farther (as a "bump") than the spinous processes of the vertebrae above. Practitioners who manipulate the spine use this bump, or *vertebra prominens,* to locate the seventh cervical vertebra.

Most people who discover this bump are not aware of its presence until neck pain or some other problem results in self-examination of the neck. In some cases, the bump becomes more apparent because of weight loss or a change in posture. Progressive weight loss could make the bump appear to be getting larger. Women whose spine begins to slump because of osteoporosis may feel that the bump has suddenly become larger.

Occasionally, a fat pad or a fatty tumor will begin to develop over the site of the bump to create a truly enlarging mass. This fatty buildup can be easily distinguished from a normal bony process, however, since the fat can be moved around, unlike a bony bump. A fatty tumor, also called a "lipoma," is harmless and benign.

In any event, a normal vertebra prominens should not be sensitive to pressure or percussion. If you have pain in this region of your spine or there is some doubt in your mind that the bump is made up of normal bone, see an orthopedic specialist for a definitive opinion.

 I have arthritis. Will taking a calcium supplement contribute to the development of spurs in my spine?

No. The spur formation in arthritis is generated by the amount of bony irritation present and not by the amount of calcium in the diet. If your diet is deficient in calcium, your body will take calcium from your bones to form the spurs caused by arthritis, thus weakening your bones. Taking extra dietary calcium, or supplementary calcium, will help protect your bones and will not stimulate or increase the development of bony spurs.

 I strained my lower pack lifting a sack of groceries out of my car. It feels as if my hip is out of place, I can't stand up straight, and one side of my back is swollen. Have I dislocated something?

Few back strains are severe enough to cause visible swelling. Generally, any apparent physical distortion is caused by spasm of the lumbar or psoas muscles, which may pull the trunk to one side or forward, causing bulging of muscles on one side of the spine. This distortion will usually disappear when you lie down and relieve the load on your spine and its supporting muscles.

If you receive a direct blow to your back and you develop a hematoma (collection of blood) or a bruise from rupture of muscle fibers and blood vessels, some visible swelling and distortion may occur along with discoloration. If this happens, put a cold pack over the injured area and see your doctor.

Q **Should I use heat or cold on a back strain?**

 A The trend these days is to use cold rather than heat when treating back problems. However, some types of problems benefit more from heat, while others respond better to cold.

Generally, when the back has been acutely injured or sprained, it's best to use cold applications the first few days. Cold will relieve pain by numbing nerves and help prevent swelling by constricting blood vessels. When there has been a direct blow to the back, causing obvious bruising, cold should *always* be applied over the injured area to reduce bleeding inside the muscles. When there is black and blue coloration, the application of heat should be delayed for four or five days.

Once pain and swelling subside, continued use of cold may delay healing by restricting blood flow. For this reason, it's usually a good idea to begin using moist heat as soon as possible to speed recovery by stimulating blood flow.

In the case of simple back strains, there may be little or no swelling in the involved joints and ligaments. Heat may then feel better, since it relaxes tight muscles. When the strain is not painful and you have only soreness and stiffness, you may use whichever feels better—heat or cold.

 Q **Will a pinched nerve in my lower back cause paralysis?**

 A When a "pinched nerve" diagnosis is made, and pain and numbness radiate down one arm or leg, many people fear that paralysis of the entire arm or leg might occur. Actually, there are several nerves supplying different portions of the extremities. Each nerve comes from a different level in the spine. When a single spinal nerve is pinched, symptoms will radiate down the arm or leg into the portion of the limb supplied by that particular nerve. If the pressure on the nerve is not relieved, the muscles supplied by that nerve will become weak and smaller and the skin may become numb. While your ability to use that arm or leg will be affected by loss of strength in the affected muscles, you'll still be able to walk or use your arm, since all the other muscles supplied by different nerves will not be affected. The worst that can happen is that isolated muscle weakness might result in weakness in an arm or a limp or foot drop (floppy foot)—which is, of course, bad enough.

Q **Can a pinched nerve cause organ failure?**

A It is a common misconception that spinal nerves control the organs of the body. Actually, the heart and other organs are supplied primarily by autonomic nerve centers that are located outside the vertebral column. There are, of course, some nerve fibers that connect the spinal nerves with the autonomic nerve centers near the vertebral column. This is why a heart attack might refer pain down your left arm and why a gall bladder problem might shoot pain up into your right shoulder area. But cutting the involved spinal nerves will not have any adverse effect on the heart or the gall bladder, since these organs have other sources of nerve supply. Even in the case of quadriplegia resulting from a severed spinal cord, the body's internal organs continue to function.

Q **Will spinal manipulation cure shingles?**

A Shingles (also called herpes zoster) is actually a viral infection in a portion of a spinal nerve (dorsal root ganglia), causing blisters and pain to appear in the portion of the skin supplied by the sensory portion of the affected nerve. This will usually disappear in a week or two, in much the same way that a fever blister on your lip disappears. The blisters of shingles, however, may leave scars.

Spinal manipulation has no effect on the course of shingles, since the condition is caused by a virus, rather than by mechanical irritation of a spinal nerve.

Q **Can my spinal curvature be corrected by manipulation?**

A If you are an adult, any spinal curvature or scoliosis you have is probably permanent. People under the age of sixteen sometimes have a curvature that can be fully or partially corrected by postural changes and other measures, such as placing a lift in one shoe. But an adult with a curvature that began in childhood has structural changes that usually make the curvature permanent.

Good posture, exercise, and other measures should be employed to combat the effects of gravity, but you cannot correct a curvature by manipulating the spine. You should not undergo a long course of spinal manipulation with the idea that you're going to change the curves in your spine. And don't worry about your curvature pinching spinal nerves. This is not likely to happen unless degenerative changes occur in discs and joints.

 Will regular exercise prevent a back injury?

 Regular exercise can be very important in preventing back trouble. Strong back muscles will not, however, guarantee protection against injury. No matter how strong your muscles are, an awkward movement can catch your back muscles off guard and result in a joint or ligament strain. If you have a structural abnormality in your spine, simple postural strain can result in irritation of unstable joints and ligaments. This is one reason people with a strong back should, like everyone else, always make a special effort to lift properly and avoid awkward strains and poor posture.

If you do all you can to keep your back muscles strong and your spine straight and you take care to avoid excessive strain and off-balance movements, your chances of having a back injury will be greatly reduced. If you keep having recurring back trouble despite observing all the proper precautions, you should have your spine examined for possible structural abnormalities.

 Why does my hip hurt if it's my back that's at fault?

When someone walks into my office complaining of "hip pain," I'm always careful to examine both the hip and the lower back. What most people refer to as their "hip" is usually an area involving their lower back. A low-back strain involving the sacroiliac joints or the lumbosacral joints at the bottom of the spine on one side is often apparent as pain on the back of the pelvis just above one buttock. A hip problem involving the hip socket is usually felt on the side of the hip and in the groin.

Movement or percussion of the lower back will usually elicit pain when the spine is involved. Hip pain can often be detected by moving the thigh around in a figure "4" fashion to see if pain occurs in the groin.

A problem involving the hip socket will often refer pain down the front of the thigh to the knee. A low-back problem, on the other hand, will sometimes refer pain through the buttock down the back of the thigh and possibly into the lower leg and foot.

You can help your doctor locate the cause of your back trouble by pointing to the area of pain and explaining which movements aggravate the pain.

Q **When I have back pain, should I rest or keep going?**

 I usually advise my patients to go by the way they feel when trying to decide how active they should be while having back trouble. Generally, pain or muscle spasm will let you know when it's time to rest your back. You should not, of course, indulge in any form of heavy exertion. Simply walking around or doing light chores is not likely to do any damage if you stop when you begin to feel uncomfortable.

Very often, moving around the house or yard is beneficial for stimulating circulation and loosening joints and muscles. As long as you feel okay, it's all right to keep going. Just remember not to push yourself when pain or muscle spasm pulls you to one side.

Some doctors routinely order patients to rest in bed for two weeks as a treatment for back pain. Enforced rest is sometimes necessary when movement causes spasm of back muscles or when severe pain radiates down one leg while standing. But there is a possibility that prolonged bed rest might actually make your back pain worse. I often see patients who have been in bed for a week or two for some problem other than back trouble and who have developed back pain while lying in bed. In these cases, arthritis or some other pre-existing problem has been aggravated by the strain placed on a sensitive spine that has been kept in one position too long.

So don't go to bed unless bed rest relieves your pain. Don't stay in bed if bed rest aggravates your back, and don't hesitate to move around if movement seems to help. Go by the way you feel. Most of the time, you won't need more than two days of bed rest.

Q **What can I do to keep my vertebrae from slipping out of place?**

A I often see patients who feel they have vertebrae that are always slipping out of place. Many of these patients believe that when their vertebrae are manipulated back into place they must move carefully in order to keep the vertebrae from slipping out of place again. Some of these apprehensive individuals are afraid to turn their head or bend over to pick up a newspaper for fear of disturbing the alignment of their spine.

Fortunately, normal, healthy spinal joints rarely slip out of place. Strong ligaments, interlocking joints, and tough disc fibers, while allowing spinal joints to move within structural barriers, make it almost impossible for a spinal joint to slip out of alignment far enough to lock itself out of place. Most often, back pain is caused by strain placed on a spinal joint that has been overloaded or made unstable by a degenerating disc or some other problem. The joint then stiffens from injury or muscle spasm, which can often be relieved by gentle loosening manipulation. Occasionally, joints become fixed or stuck together because of previous injury or from abnormal movement resulting from degenerative changes in the spine. Manipulation that restores normal movement in such joints will often result in dramatic relief of symptoms.

As a rule, spinal joints do not often slip in and out of place in such a way that they can be moved from one place to another with measured manipulation. If the joint is mobile and not locked or "stuck," the joint will automatically assume a position dictated by posture, disc thickness, joint contours, and other factors that determine how two joints fit together.

When a joint does become locked or does not move properly, simply loosening the joint with manipulation will allow the joint to return to its proper place. The key is movement. If a joint moves normally, its position and function cannot be altered by manipulation.

Some people become addicted to spinal manipulation under the false assumption that they must be manipulated regularly in order to keep their vertebrae in alignment, even though their spine is flexible and pain free. Don't become obsessed with the alignment of your vertebrae and don't be afraid to move around. *Regular exercise will actually help keep your vertebrae in alignment by keeping them mobile.*

Should I stop doing an exercise if it hurts?

 Forget about the old adage, "No pain, no gain." You should not do any exercise that causes pain.

As pain from a back injury begins to subside, you may begin walking and doing a little bending as long as it doesn't hurt. You may gradually increase the amount of exercise you do as you begin to feel better. Stop doing any exercise if it causes pain.

 What's the difference between a CAT scan, an MRI, and a bone scan?

 Computerized axial tomography (CAT or CT scan) is an imaging procedure that uses X rays beamed from different angles to produce cross-section pictures of the body. It is especially helpful in studying bones and joints and is often used in diagnosing spinal stenosis. A CAT scan requires considerable exposure to X-ray radiation.

Magnetic resonance imaging (MRI) uses magnetic fields to produce computer-generated cross-section pictures of the body. It is more effective than a CAT scan in producing soft-tissue images and is often used to diagnose disc herniation, brain tumors, and other soft tissue lesions. Since X rays are not involved in magnetic resonance, there is no harmful radiation.

A *bone scan* is a procedure in which a radioactive substance (radionuclide technetium) is injected into the body for the purpose of imaging difficult-to-detect fractures, tumors, infections, or arthritis in bones and joints. The radioactive material accumulates in damaged or cancerous bone, where it can be detected with a special imaging procedure using a Geiger counter. The amount of radiation involved in a bone scan is about equal to that of a set of lumbar spine X rays.

 How do you distinguish back trouble from kidney trouble?

 If there is mechanical-type back pain, the pain is aggravated by movement and relieved by rest. If there is pain caused by a kidney stone, there may be severe pain (often with nausea) in the back, groin, and inner thigh that is unrelieved by rest and not aggravated by movement. A person with a kidney stone cannot be still and may move about in distress, while a person with a back problem tries to avoid movement.

A constant backache unrelieved by rest and not aggravated by movement may be the result of a kidney infection if a fever is present. Always use a thermometer to take your temperature when you have constant backache, and always see your doctor when you have a fever or an unrelenting backache.

Q **How can you tell when it's time to have back surgery for a ruptured disc?**

A Surgery for a herniated disc is usually done only when a disc protrusion is pressing against a spinal nerve, causing leg pain or sciatica. It's important to remember that with or without surgery, 80 percent of patients with sciatica will eventually recover. Over 90 percent of all clinically significant nerve damage caused by disc herniation occurs in the lower back at the L4–L5 and L5–S1 levels.

When signs of nerve damage begin to appear in the arm, thigh, or leg as a result of disc herniation, as indicated by weakness, numbness, and loss of reflexes, surgery might be considered if the damage becomes progressively worse. If a "foot drop" (flopping a foot when walking) develops, surgery might be indicated. Sudden loss of bladder or bowel control, or both, during an episode of back pain may be an indication that a lumbar disc has ruptured into the spinal canal (cauda equina syndrome), indicating an immediate need for spinal surgery.

Endnotes

■

Glossary

■

Index

▪ Endnotes ▪

1. S. Bigos, O. Bowyer, G. Braen, et al. "Acute Low Back Problems in Adults." Clinical Practice Guideline No. 14. AHCPR Publication No. 95-0642. Rockville, MD: December, 1994.

2. Ibid.

3. *The Appropriateness of Spinal Manipulation for Low-Back Pain.* Rand Corporation, Santa Monica, CA: 1991–1992.

4. *Dietary Goals for the United States, Supplemental Views.* Superintendent of Documents, U.S. Government Printing Office, Washington, D.C.: November, 1977 (Dietary Guidelines for Americans, 5th edition, 2000).

5. Physicians and others who are interested in the theory underlying the practice of chiropractic should read "Finding a Good Chiropractor," Samuel Homola, D.C., *Archives of Family Medicine,* Jan/Feb, 1998, Vol. 7, No. 1, 20–23.

▪ Glossary ▪

Acupuncture. Puncturing the skin with needles at "acupoints" along channels ("meridians"). This practice is sometimes effective in relieving pain but is unproven as a method of treating illness.

Acute low back. A term used when low-back symptoms limit activity and have been present less than three months.

Acetaminophen. An over-the-counter pain reliever trademarked under the name "Tylenol." It does not have anti-inflammatory properties but is less irritating to the stomach than aspirin and other medicines used to relieve pain and inflammation.

Activator. A handheld instrument used by some chiropractors who claim they can tap "misaligned" vertebrae back into alignment, often with no evidence of misalignment.

Adjustment. A spinal manipulation used by chiropractors to realign "subluxated vertebrae."

Analgesic. Any painkilling medication, whether taken orally or applied to the skin.

Ankylosing spondylitis. A progressive inflammatory disease of the spine that causes solid bony fusion of the spinal joints.

Annulus fibrosus. The tough outer wall of a spinal disc, made up of strong crisscrossed fibers.

Anterior. The front side, as opposed to the posterior or back side.

Anti-inflammatories. Drugs and other substances used to reduce swelling and inflammation.

Applied kinesiology. An unscientific method of testing muscle strength to detect disease, vitamin deficiency, and other problems, which may then be treated with food supplements, spinal adjustments, or some other treatment method.

Arachnoiditis. Inflammation of the arachnoid membrane that covers the brain and spinal cord.

Arthritis. Inflammation of joints. There are many different kinds and causes of arthritis.

Articulation. Synonym for "joint."

Atlas. The uppermost neck vertebra, which supports the skull.

Autonomic nervous system. The part of the nervous system that controls the body's involuntary processes, such as organ function and blood pressure.

Bone scan. A scan or X ray of the skeleton taken after a radioactive dye has been injected. The dye accumulates in areas where disease or fractures may be present.

Bulging disc. Occurs when disc cartilage bulges out from between the vertebrae because of weakness in the outer wall of the disc or because of pressure from within.

Bursitis. Inflammation of the lubricating sac that surrounds a joint.

Carpal tunnel syndrome. Pain with sensory disturbance and weakness in the hand and fingers (especially in the thumb and forefinger) caused by compression of the median nerve in the wrist.

Cauda equina syndrome. Sudden weakness in the legs, numbness in the groin area, and loss of bladder or bowel control due to protrusion of a lumbar disc into the spinal canal.

Cavitation. A pop heard when joint surfaces are forcefully separated to create a vacuum that pulls in space-filling nitrogen gas.

Cervical spine. The neck part of the spine, made up of seven vertebrae.

Chelation therapy. Dubious and unsubstantiated intravenous administration of a synthetic amino acid (EDTA) to "clean out the arteries."

Chronic back pain. Back pain that lasts longer than three months.

Coccydynia. Pain in the tailbone (coccyx) area.

Coccyx. The "tailbone" at the bottom of the spine in the buttock area.

Computerized axial tomography. An X-ray imaging process that takes cross-sectional pictures of a body part. Also called a "CAT" or "CT" scan.

Contraindication. Signs or symptoms indicating that a certain diagnostic or treatment method should not be used.

D.C. Abbreviation for "Doctor of Chiropractic."

D.C.M. Abbreviation for "Doctor of Chiropractic Medicine."

D.P.T. An abbreviation for "Doctor of Physical Therapy."

Diathermy. Use of a high-frequency short wave or microwave current to generate heat deep within the tissues.

Dermatomes. Mapping of the skin to show areas supplied by certain spinal nerves.

Disc. A cartilage cushion between two vertebrae, made up of an outer portion (annulus fibrosus) and an inner portion (nucleus pulposus).

Disc degeneration. Breakdown and deterioration of disc cartilage as a result of injury, aging, or wear and tear, often called "degenerative disc disease."

Discectomy. Surgical removal of a diseased or herniated disc.

Discography. Injection of a dye into a spinal disc to determine whether the disc has a normal or abnormal configuration.

D.O. Abbreviation for "Doctor of Osteopathy."

Dura. Outer membranes covering the brain and spinal cord.

Electrodiagnostic studies. Use of electricity in nerve conduction studies and electromyography (EMG) to test nerve function.

Endorphins. Opiatelike chemicals produced in the brain to relieve perception of pain.

Epidural injection. Injection of an anesthetic or some other substance into the space just outside the dura membrane in the spinal canal.

Ergonomics. The study of proper and efficient use of the body in various environments, especially on the job and in sports.

Extension. Backward bending of the spine.

Facets. Bony surfaces that form joints between the vertebrae on the back side of the spinal column.

Fascia. A membrane or sheet of fibrous tissue that covers and separates different muscles.

Fibromyalgia. Muscle tenderness in specific spots associated with fatigue, diffuse pain, and other symptoms.

Flexion. Forward bending of the spine.

Foramen. An opening that allows a spinal nerve to pass between two vertebrae.

Fusion. A growing together of two vertebrae as a result of surgically placed bone grafts.

Galvanic stimulation. An electric current used for diagnostic and treatment purposes.

Gate control theory. A theory suggesting that spinal nerve gates can open and close due to various factors, affecting the brain's perception of pain.

Herniated disc. Extrusion or herniation of the inner portion of the disc (nucleus pulposus) through the ruptured outer wall of the disc (annulus fibrosus). (*See* "Ruptured disc.")

Homeopathy. An unproven method of healing that uses highly diluted solutions made from substances that cause the same symptoms as the disease being treated.

Hydrotherapy. Use of water in a treatment, as in a whirlpool.

Imaging study. Any study, such as an X ray or a CT scan, that produces images of the body part being studied.

Intermittent claudication. Leg cramps that occur as a result of circulatory insufficiency after walking a certain distance. The cramps disappear when walking stops and then recur when walking resumes.

Invasive treatment. Any procedure that involves penetrating the skin.

Iontophoresis. The movement of ions in solution from one electrode to another by a direct current, as in the electrical transfer of chemical substances into the body with a galvanic current

"Killer subluxations." Allegedly misaligned or malfunctioning vertebrae that some chiropractors claim can cause fatal illness.

Kinesiology. Study of the anatomy and mechanics of movement. Not to be confused with "applied kinesiology," an unscientific method of muscle testing. (*See* "Applied kinesiology.")

Kyphosis. An abnormal curve of the thoracic spine producing a hump in the upper back.

Lamina. Structures on the back side of a vertebra contributing to the formation of a spinal canal that encases the spinal cord.

Laminectomy. Removal of the lamina on the back side of a vertebra in order to relieve pressure on the spinal cord and spinal nerves.

Lateral bending. Bending of the spine to one side or the other.

Ligament. Tough, fibrous tissue that connects and hold joints together.

L.M.T. An abbreviation for "Licensed Massage Therapist."

Lumbar lordosis. An exaggerated lumbar curve that produces a sway back.

Lumbar spine. The lower part of the back, made up of five lumbar vertebrae.

Lumbar support. A wraparound corset that supports the lumbar spine by encircling the trunk from the waist down.

Lumbosacral joints. The joints connecting the lumbar spine with the sacrum at the base of the spine, the most common site of back pain.

Lumbosacral sprain/strain. Low-back pain following injury to muscles, joints, or ligaments in the lumbosacral area of the spine.

Magnetic Resonance Imaging (MRI). A method of imaging that uses the energy of a magnetic field to obtain cross-sectional pictures of body structures. No radiation is involved.

Maintenance care. Treatment offered by some chiropractors who believe that regular spinal adjustments will maintain health and prevent disease, sometimes called "preventive-maintenance care."

Manipulation. Manual movement of bones and joints to relieve stiffness or locking of joints and to restore mobility.

Massage therapist. A licensed practitioner who provides complementary therapeutic massage for musculoskeletal problems.

Mixer chiropractor. A chiropractor who uses physical therapy and other treatment methods along with manipulation of the spine.

Modality. Any one of a number of passive treatment methods used in physical therapy, such as ultrasound, electrical stimulation, or massage.

M.P.T. An abbreviation for "Master's Degree in Physical Therapy."

Muscle spasm. Painful, involuntary contraction of muscles.

Musculoskeletal system. Pertaining to muscles and skeletal joints.

Myelogram. Injection of a dye into the spinal canal before back surgery so that structures, such as a herniated disc, can be located and better visualized with an X ray or a CT scan.

Myositis. Inflammation of muscle fibers.

Myofascitis. Inflammation of muscles and their surrounding fascial sheaths.

Myotome. A group of muscles supplied by a single spinal nerve.

Nerve root. A nerve that exits the spinal canal by passing through an opening (foramen) between two vertebrae.

Nerve conduction studies. Testing peripheral nerves by stimulating the nerve at one point and measuring its conduction of sensory and motor function at another point.

Neurogenic claudication. Leg pain and weakness that occurs while standing, usually caused by spinal stenosis (narrowing of the spinal canal) and usually relieved by sitting or by bending forward.

Neurologic deficit. Loss of strength, sensation, or tendon reflexes as a result of damage to the nervous system or a spinal nerve.

Neurologist. A physician trained in the diagnosis and nonsurgical treatment of nervous system problems.

Neuromuscular. Pertaining to nerves and muscles.

Neurosurgeon. A physician who specializes in surgical treatment of problems affecting the nervous system, such as a herniated disc or a brain tumor.

Nocebo effect. An adverse reaction resulting from a patient's fear and expectation that a medication, a treatment, or lack of treatment will result in illness.

Nucleus pulposus. The inner gelatinous portion of a spinal disc.

Objective symptoms. Symptoms that can be observed and measured by a physician.

Opiates. Pain-relieving narcotics that contain opium or one of its derivatives.

Orthopedist. A surgeon trained in the treatment of skeletal problems, such as fractures, scoliosis, torn muscles, or dislocated joints.

Osteomalacia. Bone softening caused by a deficiency in vitamin D and inadequate mineralization of new bone.

Osteopath. A physician trained in use of manipulative treatment along with standard medical care.

Osteopenia. Early demineralization of bone, often a precursor to osteoporosis.

Osteophyte. A projecting overgrowth of bone, often called a "spur."

Osteoporosis. Advanced demineralization that results in brittle bones that are easily fractured. "Crush fractures" in the thoracic spine are commonly caused by osteoporosis.

Paraphysiological space. The point reached when a joint is forcefully and passively moved beyond its normal, active range of motion.

Parasympathetic nervous system. A set of autonomic nerves that works along with the sympathetic nervous system in controlling the body's automatic or involuntary functions.

Pars interarticularis. An arch or bridge of bone connecting the body of a vertebra to the joints on each side.

Physiatrist. A physician who specializes in the care of musculoskeletal problems, focusing on physical treatment methods and rehabilitation.

Physical therapist. Practitioners with an RPT certification (registered physical therapist) who work in the field of physical medicine and rehabilitation, usually under a physician's prescription. Thirty-five states now allow direct access to a physical therapist for evaluation and treatment without a physician's referral.

Placebo. An inactive or make-believe medicine often used to compare with the effects of a real treatment method. A placebo, such as a sugar pill, can have a beneficial effect if the patient believes in the "medicine."

Primary-care provider. A health-care professional who provides basic health services, manages routine health-care needs, and is usually the first contact when someone needs care.

Pseudoscience. An unsubstantiated theory that is represented as being scientific but is supported by false information.

Psoas muscles. Muscles that attach between the transverse processes of vertebrae and a bony prominence at the top of the femur (thigh bone). Contraction of these muscles to flex the hips will sometimes aggravate back pain by pulling on the lower spine.

Psychosomatic. When signs and symptoms of illness appear because of stress, fear of disease, or psychological problems.

Quackery. Deliberate use of misinformation to promote unsubstantiated and scientifically implausible treatment methods.

Radiculitis. Inflammation or irritation of a spinal nerve root, resulting in symptoms referred into the part of the body supplied by the nerve.

Radiculopathy. Pain, weakness, loss of sensation, diminished reflexes, and other symptoms caused by damage to a nerve root, most often the result of disc herniation or spur formation.

Radiograph. A medical term for an image on X-ray film.

Radiologist. A specialist trained in the use of radiation for diagnosing and treating disease. Radiologists commonly evaluate X-ray films for other practitioners.

Range of motion. Joint movement measured in degrees in all directions.

Referred pain. Pain felt in a part of the body remote from its actual source.

Reflex. An involuntary response to a stimulus, as in tapping a tendon to determine if the muscle involved is receiving adequate nerve supply.

Reflex sympathetic dystrophy. Pain, sweating, decreased skin temperature, and other autonomic changes in an extremity as a result of injury to bone and soft tissue.

Reflexology. An unproven diagnostic and treatment method based on belief that each body part is represented on the hands and feet and that pressing or massaging certain spots on the hands and soles of the feet will have therapeutic effects in other parts of the body.

Rheumatologist. A physician who specializes in the diagnosis and treatment of arthritis and other inflammatory diseases involving muscles and joints.

Rheumatoid arthritis (RA). An autoimmune disease that erodes joints and supporting tissues.

Roentgenology. The science of using X rays for diagnostic purposes.

Ruptured disc. A break or tear in the outer wall of a disc, predisposing to disc herniation. (*See* "Herniated disc.")

Sacroiliac (SI) joints. Joints that hold the sacrum and the pelvis together, one on each side. The sacroiliac joints can be found by locating the dimple above each buttock.

Sacroiliac support. A strap or belt wrapped tightly around the pelvis to support the sacroiliac joints.

Sacrum. A triangular bone that forms the base of the spinal column and joins the pelvis on each side. Important spinal nerves supplying voluntary control of bladder and anal muscles are protected in their passage through solid bony openings in the sacrum.

Saddle anesthesia. Loss of sensation in the skin over the perineum (the area between the anus and the genitals), usually as a result of a disc protrusion into the spinal canal.

Sciatica. Leg pain that originates from lower lumbar and sacral nerves that pass through the buttock area and down the back of the thigh into the lower leg and foot.

Scoliosis. Abnormal curves of the spine from side to side, forming an s-shaped curvature. In an adult, such curvatures are structural and cannot be corrected.

Spinal adjustment. A chiropractic treatment using the hands or an instrument to "realign subluxated vertebrae."

Spinal canal. A tunnel formed by the openings in stacked vertebrae for the purpose of housing and protecting the spinal cord.

Spinal manipulation. Manual therapy to loosen a locked or stiff spine.

Spinal stenosis. Narrowing of the spinal canal to such a degree that there may be some encroachment upon the spinal cord and its nerves.

Spinous processes. The bony projections that form bumps on the back of the vertebrae. Practitioners who manipulate the spine use these bumps to locate vertebrae and for leverage in the use of manipulation.

Spondylitis. Inflammation of vertebrae, most often as a result of aging and wear and tear.

Spondylolisthesis. Progressive, forward slipping of one vertebra over another, often as a result of a congenital defect in joint structures, usually the pars articularis. A limited amount of forward slipping sometimes occurs as a result of degenerative changes in joints and discs.

Spondylosis. Degenerative changes in the joints and discs of the spine that are common (but not alarming) changes associated with aging.

Spondylolysis. A defect, resembling a crack or a fracture, in the pars articularis that may allow one vertebra to slip forward over the vertebra below, especially when disc cartilage begins to weaken and deteriorate with aging or wear and tear.

Straight chiropractor. A chiropractor who believes that misaligned vertebrae cause most illnesses and that spinal adjustment is the only treatment needed.

Straight leg raise (SLR). A test in which one leg is raised straight up to stretch the sciatic nerve to determine if pain at a certain elevation indicates compression or entrapment of a branch of the sciatic nerve.

Stroke. Sudden loss of brain function caused by blockage or rupture of a blood vessel supplying the brain.

Subjective symptoms. Symptoms felt and expressed by the patient but not detectable by physical examination.

Subluxation. A medical term for partial and often painful dislocation of a joint, which is not the same as an asymptomatic "chiropractic subluxation" (a slight misalignment that many chiropractors believe is a cause of disease).

Surface electromyography (SEMG). An unsubstantiated procedure that attempts to locate "chiropractic subuxations" by measuring skin temperature and electrical activity in muscles around the spine. This procedure is not the same as needle electromyography, a legitimate neurologic test in which needles are inserted into muscles to locate nerve damage.

Sympathetic nervous system. A set of autonomic nerves that control involuntary functions.

Tendon. A strong fibrous cord that attaches a muscle to a bone.

Thermography. A procedure that uses infrared heat to record images generated by the heat in skin and muscles. It has little diagnostic value except in special cases where circulation and skin temperature are affected by nerve injury, as in reflex sympathetic dystrophy. It will not locate subluxations as claimed by some chiropractors.

Thoracic spine. The upper part of the spine between the shoulder blades, consisting of twelve vertebrae. Sometimes called the dorsal spine.

Thoracic outlet syndrome. Vascular and neurologic symptoms in an arm as a result of pressure on blood vessels and nerve fibers at some point between the base of the neck and the armpit, often the result of a cervical rib or an abnormal (scalenus) neck muscle.

Traction. Stretching applied along the axis of the spine to relieve muscle tension and decompress spinal discs. This is sometimes used to relieve compression on a spinal nerve.

Transcutaneous electrical nerve stimulation (TENS). A small battery-operated device that provides electrical stimulation through electrodes applied over the skin for the purpose of relieving pain by modifying pain perception.

Transverse process. Projection of bone on each side of a vertebra where muscles are attached. Transverse processes are commonly used as contact points and levers in the performance of spinal manipulation.

Ultrasound. The use of high frequency sound waves to generate heat beneath the surface of the skin. Sometimes used to break up calcium formations in the body. Sound waves have been used to push medication through the skin in a process called "iontophoresis."

Vertebra and vertebrae. Vertebra is a bone of the spine, made up of a vertebral body, two transverse processes, and one spinous process. Vertebrae is the plural form of the word vertebra.

Vertebral artery. Arteries, one on each side, that thread up through holes in the transverse processes of cervical vertebrae to supply the brain with blood.

Vertebral subluxation complex. The newest definition of a "chiropractic subluxation," suggesting that changes in nerve, muscle, connective, and vascular tissues indicate the presence of "kinesiologic aberrations of spinal articulations" (subluxations) that are not detectable by X-ray examination but which can "compromise neural integrity and may influence organ system function and general health."

Viscera. The internal organs of the body, especially those contained within the thoracic and abdominal cavities.

Vitalism. The concept that the functions of the body are due to a "life force" that cannot be explained by the laws of physics and chemistry. Chiropractors refer to this force as "Innate Intelligence," which they feel will heal the body if spinal adjustments are used to remove "nerve interference" hindering the healing process.

X ray. A radiant energy in the form of a ray that passes through the body to form an image on film.

▪ Index ▪

A

abdominal exercise, 168–170, 206–207
acupuncture, 251
Agency for Healthcare Research and Quality, 1, 21, 121–122, 262
aging, and back pain, 240–247; and exercise, 245–246; and leg pain, 24; and neck pain, 60; and posture, 209; and sex, 233
alcohol, 39, 161
American Chiropractic Association, 62
American Journal of Public Health, 76
amines, 39, 51
ankle tendons, tight, 125–126, 138
ankylosing spondylitis, 182, 183, 193–196, 217
arm pain. *See* pain, arm
arteries, hardening, 24
artery blockage, 23–24
arthritis, 182–202; ankylosing spondylitis, 182, 183, 193–196, 217; and calcium, 269; home treatment, 188; osteoarthritis, 182, 183, 185–190; and posture, 205; rheumatoid arthritis, 182, 183, 190–193; shoulder, 13, 66; and sleep, 200–201
arthritis, gouty. *See* gout
aspirin, 184–185, 200–201. *See also* medication

B

back pain. *See* pain, back
back strain, 76–78
back support, 84–85, 117
bed rest, 78–79, 217–218, 273
bladder dysfunction, 16, 76, 264. *See also* cauda equina syndrome

blood clot, 23–24
body mass index (BMI), 155–156
bone scan, 275
bowel dysfunction, 76, 264. *See also* cauda equina syndrome
Buerger's disease, 24
bursitis, 13, 66

C

caffeine, 31, 38
calcium, and aging, 245; and arthritis, 269; and osteoporosis, 105–110; requirements, 108; sources of, 106–108, 109, 110; supplements, 107–110
calorie, intake, 154–155; reduction, 142; requirements, 153–157; sample diet plans, 158–160
cancer, 11, 20, 40, 243; and back pain, 78; colon, 47, 49; prostate, 15
carbohydrates, 49–50, 144–148, 163
carpal tunnel syndrome, 13, 71–73, 74, 219
CAT scan, 19, 275
cauda equina syndrome, 86, 90, 117, 241–242
Centers for Disease Control and Prevention, 1
cervical collar, 55–56
cervical pillows, 58–59
cervical traction, 63–65
chairs, selection, 210–212
chemonucleosis (chymopapain injection), 257
children, and back pain, 255–256
chiropractor, 250, 254–256, 259–266; mixed, 259–260; payment, 264–265; selecting, 123, 261–266; subluxation-based, 259–261
chymopapain injection, 21, 257
cigarettes, 31, 38, 76

circulatory problems, 23–24

cluster headache, 8, 9, 30, 37, 50; and diet, 41–42; medication, 51

Composition of Foods: Raw, Processed, Prepared, 158

computerized axial tomography. *See* CAT scan

constipation, 46–50; and back pain, 46–47, 84; causes of, 48–49; and colon cancer, 47; and laxatives, 48–49

cortisone, and osteoporosis, 111

cracking joints, 120–122, 136–138, 262

crutches, and back pain, 83

cryotherapy (cold), 83, 251, 270; for neck pain, 56

curvature, spinal, 96–100, 118, 271–272

D

depression, 255

diathermy, 115, 251

diet, 140–163; and alcohol, 161; and arthritis, 184; balanced, 145–147, 157–158; body mass index (BMI), 155–156; and calcium, 105–110, 163; calorie reduction, 142; calorie requirements, 153–157; carbohydrates, 49–50, 144–148, 163; and constipation, 49–50; fats, 146, 150–151, 160; fiber, 49–50, 147–148; food groups, 145–147, 163; food preparation, 161–163; and gout, 197; and headaches, 41–42; ideal weight, 153; natural foods, 160–161; and osteoporosis, 105–110, 245; sample meal plans, 151–152, 158–160

Dietary Goals for the United States, 140, 144, 146, 148

Dietary Guidelines for Americans, 140, 144, 161

dieting, 141–142, 147, 148, 163. *See also* diet; weight loss

disc, herniated, 85–87, 90, 117, 264; and aging, 241–242; and sex, 235; surgery, 276; treatment, 60

disc, ruptured, 90, 92

disc, slipped, 89–90

diverticulitis, 47, 49

doctors, 61, 79, 80; selection of, 16–18. *See also* specialists

"dowager's hump." *See* osteoporosis

E

elbow pain. *See* pain, elbow

electrical stimulation, 115, 251

epicondylitis (tennis elbow), 70

ergonomics, 218–220

exercise, 115, 124, 137, 181, 275; abdominal, 168–170, 206–207; and aging, 245–246; ankle tendons, 125–126; and ankylosing spondylitis, 195–196; and arthritis, 184; back, 129, 165–168, 170–174, 176–177; frequency, 179–180; full body, 175–176; hamstrings, 126–127; and headaches, 43–44; hip flexors, 127–129, 169; leg strengthening, 174–175; neck, 136–137; and osteoarthritis, 189–190; and osteoporosis, 112–113; and postural kyphosis (hump back), 177–178; and pregnancy, 224; and rheumatoid arthritis, 192–193; rib cage muscles, 129–130; shoulder, 67–69; side muscles, 129; and swayback, 179; thigh bands, 127; vertebrae-loosening, 130–136; in water, 177; and weight loss, 143–144

F

facet syndrome, 100

family practice physician, 249, 250, 252

fiber, 49–50, 147–148

fibromyalgia, 114, 198–199

fomentation roll (moist heat), 33

food groups, 145–147, 163

food pyramid, 146–147

foot care, 207–208

foot drop, 20, 21, 26, 276

G

Gedosh, E.A., *xiii*
glandular disease, 20–21
gout, 13, 71, 184, 196–198
Gray's Anatomy, 96
Guidelines to Acute Low Back Problems in Adults, 115

H

hamstrings, short, 125, 126–127, 138, 208
headache, causes of, 6–7, 38–43, 44–47, 51; chronic, 31; diagnosis of, 7, 10; and diet, 41–42; and exercise, 43–44; medication, 51; remedies, 31–38; and tension, 7, 30, 50; types of, 7–8, 9–10, 50. *See also* cluster headache; migraine
heat, fomentation roll, 33; for neck pain, 56; versus cold therapy, 57–58, 83, 270
herniated disc. *See* disc, herniated
hip flexors, 127–129, 138, 169, 170
hip pain. *See* pain, hip
hydrotherapy, 251
hypoglycemia, 38, 44–46, 51

I

intermittent claudication, 24
internists, 253
inverse traction, 95–96

J

Jacobson technique, 36
joints, cracking, 120–122, 136, 262
Journal of the American Medical Association, 85

K

kidney infection, 7–8, 15, 276
kidney stones, 15, 243–244, 275
"kissing spine," 103
kyphoplasty, 105

L

laminectomy, 257
laxatives, 48–49
leg pain. *See* pain, leg
lifting, 212–214
lipoma, 269
lumbago, 199
lumbar pain. *See* pain, back
lumbar support, 84–85, 117
lupus, 201–202

M

magnetic resonance imaging (MRI), 19, 20, 275
manipulation, 73, 90, 249, 251, 253; cervical (neck), 35, 62–63, 73, 135–137, 191; cracking joints, 121, 122; and osteoarthritis, 189; and scoliosis, 99; and shingles, 271; and slipped disc, 89–90; spinal 21–22, 115–116, 262, 265, 266, 267, 274; and spinal curvature, 271–272
Marie-Strumpell disease. *See* ankylosing spondylitis
massage, 57, 73, 251; back, 137–138; neck, 33–34
mattress, 215; and arthritis, 200–201; and back pain, 80–81
medical tests, 17, 19, 20
medication, 116–117, 245–246; for arthritis, 184–185, 200–201; for back pain, 77; and constipation, 84; for headaches, 51
meningitis, 7
menopause, 21, 104, 106, 234, 244

migraine, 6, 50; medication, 51; symptoms, 8–9, 30; treatment, 37, 41–42
monosodium glutamate (MSG), 31–38, 40–41, 51
MRI (magnetic resonance imaging), 19, 20
myofascitis, 198–199

N

National Academy of Sciences, 108
National Council Against Health Fraud, 62
neck cracking, 139
neck "crick," 10, 53, 54–60, 73, 199. *See also* pain, neck
neck massage, 33–34
neck pain. *See* pain, neck
nerve, pinched, 23, 73, 263–264, 270–271; tests for, 87–89; treatment, 60–61
neurogenic claudication, 24
neurologist, 250, 251–252
nicotine, 31, 38, 76
nitrites, 39–40, 51; and headaches, 31

O

Occupational Medicine, 76
orthopedist, 250, 252
osteoarthritis, 185–190
osteomalacia, 104
osteopaths, 250, 254
osteoporosis, 103–114, 118, 244–245; and aging, 105; and calcium, 105–110; and cortisone, 111; and diet, 105–110; and exercise, 112–113; prevention, 105–110

P

Paget's disease, 24, 187
pain, arm, 13–14, 29, 74
pain, back, 1, 2, 75–85, 90–92, 94–96, 103; and aging, 240–247; and bed rest, 217–218, 273; and bedding, 80–82; and body weight, 143–144, 163; and cancer, 78, 243; causes, 14–15, 19; in children, 255–256; chronic, 75, 116; and constipation, 46–47, 84; and crutches, 83; and depression, 255; and foot care, 207–208; heat versus cold therapy, 57, 58, 83, 270; and hip flexors, 127–129; and kidney problems, 7–8, 15, 243–244, 275, 276; and osteoporosis, 244–245; postpartum, 226–228; and posture, 203, 204–212; and pregnancy, 222–230; prevention, 122; and sex, 234–239; and sleeping postures, 214–218; and stress, 114–115, 118; surgery, 257, 276; and tension myositis syndrome, 255; treatments, 115; types, 25–28
pain, elbow, 13, 69–71, 74
pain, hand, 71–73
pain, hip, 19, 29, 272–273
pain, leg, 19, 23, 24, 90–92, 94–96, 116; and aging, 240–247; and blood clots, 23–24; and disc herniation, 86–87; traction, 82–83, 92, 94–96
pain, neck, 10–11, 29, 53–65, 199; causes, 54; manipulation, 35, 62–63, 73, 135–137, 191; and pillows, 58–60, 73; and pinched nerves, 60–61; treatment, 54–60
pain, radiating, 5, 19, 73, 187, 242
pain, shoulder, 12–13, 29, 66–69, 74
pain, wrist, 13, 71–73; and carpal tunnel syndrome, 74, 219
paralysis, 270–271
pelvic harness traction, 92, 94
pelvic tilt, 208–209
percutaneous discectomy, 21, 257
percutaneous vertebroplasty, 105
phosphorus, and osteoporosis, 105–106
physiatrists, 249, 252–253
physical therapists, 250, 256–257
physical therapy, 251
physicians, 61, 79, 80; selection, 16–18. *See also* specialists
pillows, 73; and back pain, 81–82; cervical, 58–59; selection, 58–60
pinched nerve. *See* nerve, pinched
poker spine. *See* ankylosing spondylitis

polymyalgia rheumatica, 198–199
polymyositis, 198–199
postural hypotension (dizziness), 218
postural kyphosis (hump back); and exercise,
   177–178
posture, 98, 180; and aging, 209; and
   ankylosing spondylitis, 194–195; and back
   pain, 203, 204–212; and ergonomics,
   218–220; and sitting, 209–212; and sleep,
   214–218
pregnancy, and back pain, 222–230; and back
   support, 228–229; and exercise, 224; and
   sex, 233–234, 238
prevention, back pain, 122
prostate, 15

R

radiculitis, 60
radiculopathy, 91, 116
radiology, 253
Raynaud's disease, 73
rehabilitation, 251
relaxation, 36–37
rheumatoid arthritis, 13, 182, 183, 190–193
rheumatologists, 253–254
Rolfing (massage), 137–138

S

salt, 41; and osteoporosis, 106
sciatic pain (sciatica), 19–20, 76, 77, 215; and
   herniated disc, 85, 241, 242; medication,
   116; tests, 89
scoliosis, 96–100, 206, 271–272
self-help, for arthritis, 188; for headaches,
   31–38; for leg pain, 82–83; spinal
   adjustment, 134–136
sex, 231–239; and arthritis, 200; and back
   pain, 234–239; benefits of, 232–233; and
   menopause, 234; and pregnancy, 233–234,
   238
sexual positions, 236–238

shingles, 271
shoe lifts, 99–100
shoulder pain. See pain, shoulder
sitting, 209–212
sleeping postures, 214–218
smoking, and back pain, 76; and headache,
   31, 38
sodium, 41; and osteoporosis, 106
sodium nitrites, 31, 39–40, 41
specialists, 17; chiropractors, 250, 254–256,
   259–266; family practice, 249, 250, 252;
   internists, 253; neurologists, 250, 251–252;
   orthopedists, 250, 252; osteopaths, 250,
   254; physiatrists, 249, 252–253; physical
   therapists, 250, 256–257; radiologists, 253;
   rheumatologists, 253–254; selection,
   248–258
spinal abnormalities, 96–103
spinal adjustment, home, 134–136
spinal arthritis, 189–202
spinal curvature, 96–100, 206, 271–272
spinal fusion, 257. See also surgery
spinal manipulation. See manipulation
spinal stenosis, 24
spine, diagram of, 18
spondylolisthesis, 100–102
strain, back, 76–78
stress, 118; and back pain, 114–115; and
   headaches, 42
stretching, back, 129; neck, 35–36, 63–65
support, back, 84–85, 117
surgery, 21–23, 61, 257, 276
swayback, 179
swelling, 269
systemic lupus erythematosus, 201

T

temporal arteritis, 8, 198
tendonitis, 66, 68–69, 70
tennis elbow, 13, 70
tension myositis syndrome, 255
thermography, 122, 261, 262
thigh bands, tight, 127, 138

tobacco. *See* smoking

traction, 251; cervical, 63–65; inverse, 95–96; leg, 82–83, 90–92, 94–96; lower back, 92, 94–96; neck, 35–36, 73; pelvic harness, 92, 94

transcutaneous electrical stimulation (TENS), 251

transitional vertebra, 102

treatment, types of, 251

Type M disorders, 6, 25–28

Type O disorders, 6, 29

U

ultrasound, 115, 251

urinary stone, 15

U.S. Department of Agriculture, 146, 161

U.S. Department of Health and Human Services, 115

U.S. Public Health Service, 1

V

vertebra prominens, 268, 269

vertebrae, cervical, 61; and cracking joints, 120–122, 136, 262; diagram, 18; loosening

exercises, 130–136; misalignments, 262–263, 274; neck, 136, 137, 268, 269; slipping, 274

vitamin C, sources of, 93

W

weight loss, 92, 141–142, 148–151; and calorie intake, 154–155; and gout, 197–198; and osteoarthritis, 189

weight ranges, 155

wrist pain. *See* pain, wrist

X

X rays, 20, 26–30, 121–122, 262

More Hunter House Books on
Health, Healing & Sexuality

THE ART OF GETTING WELL: A Five-Step Plan for Maximizing Health When You Have a Chronic Illness *by* David Spero, R.N.

Self-management programs have become a key way for people to deal with chronic illness. Spero brings together the medical, psychological, and spiritual aspects of getting well in a five-step approach that asks you to slow down and use your energy for the things that matter; make small changes that build self-confidence; get help and nourish your social ties; value your body and treat it with affection and respect; and take responsibility for getting the best care you can.

224 pages ... Paperback $15.95 ... Hardcover $25.95

CHINESE HERBAL MEDICINE MADE EASY: Natural and Effective Remedies for Common Illnesses *by* Thomas Richard Joiner

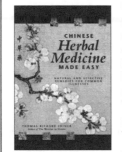

Chinese herbal medicine is an ancient system for maintaining health and prolonging life. This book demystifies the subject, with clear explanations and easy-to-read alphabetical listings of more than 750 herbal remedies for over 250 common illnesses ranging from acid reflux and AIDS to breast cancer, pain management, sexual dysfunction, and weight loss. Whether a newcomer to herbology or a seasoned practitioner, you will find this book a valuable addition to your health library.

432 pages ... Paperback $24.95 ... Hardcover $34.95

MAKING LOVE BETTER THAN EVER: Reaching New Heights of Passion and Pleasure After 40 by Barbara Keesling, Ph.D.

Great sex is not reserved for those under forty. With maturity comes the potential for a soulful loving that draws on all we are to deepen our ties of intimacy and nurturing. That is the loving that sustains relationships into later years. In this book, Dr. Barbara Keesling shows couples how to reignite sexual feelings while reconnecting emotionally. She provides relaxation and body-image exercises that heighten sexual response, reduce anxiety, improve body image, and promote playfulness and spontaneity.

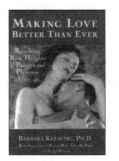

208 pp. ... 14 b/w photos ... Paperback $13.95 ... Hardcover $24.95

To order or for our FREE catalog call (800) 266-5592

More Hunter House Books on
Fitness, Exercise & Health

GET FIT WHILE YOU SIT: Easy Workouts from Your Chair
by Charlene Torkelson

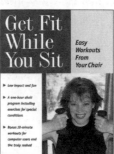

Here is a total-body workout that can be done right from your chair, anywhere. It is perfect for office workers, travelers, and those with movement limitations. The *One-Hour Chair Program* is a full-body, low-impact workout that includes light aerobics and exercises to be done with or without weights. The *5-Day Short Program* features five compact workouts for those short on time, and the *Ten-Minute Miracles* is a group of easy exercises perfect for anyone on the go.

160 pages ... 212 b/w photos ... Paperback $12.95 ... Hardcover $22.95

SHAPEWALKING: Six Easy Steps to Your Best Body
by Marilyn Bach, Ph.D., and Lorie Schleck, M.A., P.T. ... *2nd Edition*

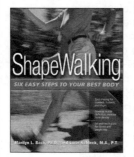

Millions of Americans want an easy, low-cost approach to total fitness. *ShapeWalking* is the answer—a program that includes aerobic exercise, strength training, and flexibility stretching and is suited for exercisers of all levels.

ShapeWalking is ideal for people who want to control weight, develop muscle definition, prevent or reverse loss of bone density, and spot-shape the stomach, buttocks, arms, and thighs. This all-new second edition includes over 70 black-and-white photographs and updated exercises and resources.

160 pages ... 70 photos ... Paperback $14.95 ... Hardcover $24.95 ... SEPTEMBER 2002

SELF-HELP FOR HYPERVENTILATION SYNDROME: Recognizing and Correcting Your Breathing Pattern Disorder
by Dinah Bradley ... *3rd Edition*

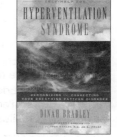

Chronic hyperventilation especially affects asthmatics, premenstrual and menopausal women, overachievers, and workaholics. Symptoms include breathlessness, chest pains, palpitations, broken sleep, stomach or bowel problems, dizziness, and anxiety. This book explains causes and symptoms and presents a well-tested program that the author has developed for readers to use in order to break the hyperventilation cycle and breathe freely again.

128 pages ... Paperback $12.95 ... Hardcover $22.95

Order online at www.hunterhouse.com ... or see last page

More Hunter House Books on
Fitness & Exercise

pg. 3

FUSION FITNESS: Combining the Best from East and West
by Chan Ling Yap, Ph.D.

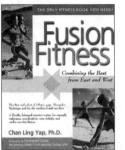

Here is the next step in fitness programs, a combination of the best Western and Eastern techniques including Pilates, Alexander Technique, Callanetics, yoga, and T'ai Chi used to create a dynamic fitness program for strength, endurance, toning, coordination, core stability, and cardiovascular fitness. The author explains how the different techiniques have been combined and, in some cases, used to create new exercises. The book has over 130 photos and illustrations.

224 pages ... 62 photos ... 70 b/w illus. ... Paperback $15.95 ... OCTOBER 2002

THE COMPLETE GUIDE TO JOSEPH H. PILATES' TECHNIQUES OF PHYSICAL CONDITIONING: Applying the Principles of Body Control
by Allen Menezes, Founder of the Pilates Institute of Australasia

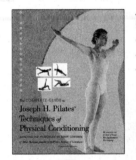

Almost 80 years ago, Joseph Pilates developed a bodywork system, wildly popular today, focusing on strengthening the core muscles of the abdomen and strengthening and increasing flexibility in the arms and legs. This guide to Pilates' techniques includes a complete floor program of basic, intermediate, and advanced routines, with detailed descriptions of each exercise and step-by-step photographs. There is a special section on relieving back, ankle, and shoulder pain, and insights on how Pilates work can be adapted by athletes.

208 pages ... 191 b/w photos ... 80 illus. & charts ... Paperback $19.95 ... Spiral Bound $26.95

PEAK PERFORMANCE FITNESS: Maximizing Your Fitness Potential Without Injury or Strain *by* Jennifer Rhodes, M.S.PT

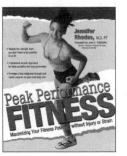

Jennifer Rhodes looks at the body as an integrated system and offers a step-by-step plan for developing cardiovascular capacity, strength, and flexibility. In a friendly, vibrant style she discusses the purpose of each exercise and how it works to improve the body's overall functioning.

The book includes several real-life success stories, and detailed photographs and anatomical drawings to illustrate the exercises.

160 pages ... 46 b/w photos ... 31 illus. ... Paperback $14.95

To order or for our FREE catalog call (800) 266-5592

ORDER FORM

10% DISCOUNT on orders of $50 or more —
20% DISCOUNT on orders of $150 or more —
30% DISCOUNT on orders of $500 or more —
On cost of books for fully prepaid orders

NAME

ADDRESS

CITY/STATE   ZIP/POSTCODE

PHONE   COUNTRY (outside of U.S.)

TITLE	QTY	PRICE	TOTAL
Chiropractor's Self-Help ... Book (paper)		@ $17.95	
Chiropractor's Self-Help ... Book (cloth)		@ $29.95	

Prices subject to change without notice

Please list other titles below:

		@ $	
		@ $	
		@ $	
		@ $	
		@ $	

Check here to receive our book catalog ☐   *FREE*

Shipping Costs:
By Priority Mail, first book $4.50, each additional book $1.00
By UPS and to Canada, first book $5.50, each additional book $1.50
For rush orders and other countries call us at (510) 865-5282

TOTAL
Less discount @ _____ %   (_____)
TOTAL COST OF BOOKS
Calif. residents add 7½ sales tax
add Shipping & handling
TOTAL ENCLOSED
Please pay in U.S. funds only

☐ Check   ☐ Money Order   ☐ Visa   ☐ MasterCard   ☐ Discover

Card # _____ Exp. date _____

Signature _____

Complete and mail to:

Hunter House Inc., Publishers
PO Box 2914, Alameda CA 94501-0914
Phone (510) 865-5282 Fax (510) 865-4295
You can also order by calling **(800) 266-5592**
of from **www.hunterhouse.com**

CBB 8/2002